Praise for Christine Avanti's
Skinny Chicks Don't Eat Salads

"Christine knows how to get her clients in the best shape of their lives. Her nutrition knowledge is tops and she has given me wonderful advice on how to maintain my body."

—Samantha Harris, TV host, *Dancing with the Stars* and *The Insider*

"At *E! News* we go to Christine Avanti as our number one nutrition and weight loss expert. She is always tapped into the hottest trends in health, diet, and weight loss."

—Giuliana Rancic, *E! News* host, costar of Style Network's *Giuliana & Bill*

"After years of struggling with the obsessive pursuit of getting skinny and the pressures of the entertainment industry, I finally feel healthy, happy, and full of energy. Christine Avanti's program has changed my life."

—Lisa Germani, director of talent, TV Guide Network

"Christine has put together a nutritional program that is effective and easy to follow. Kudos Christine, I wish I had published it first."

—Jason Diamond, MD, FACS, board-certified plastic surgeon, featured on E! Network's *Dr. 90210*

"Christine Avanti has written a medically sound and practical guide to losing weight and getting fit. Chock-full of advice and recipes, *Skinny Chicks* sets the standard for fitness and good health."

—J. Ron Eaker, MD, FACOG, author of *Fat-Proof Your Family* and *A Woman's Guide to Hormone Health*, clinical advisor to the American Running Association

"We can always count on Christine Avanti when it comes to weight loss and nutrition. Her information is always fun, fresh, and cutting edge."

—Maureen Heaton, *E! News*

"Avanti is wise, experienced, practical, and medically sensible. *Skinny Chicks* is not only for skinny-chick wannabes—it also works for the guys who love them."

—Marc Siegel, MD, associate professor of medicine at the New York University School of Medicine, Fox News medical contributor, *LA Times* columnist

"Unlike short-term fad diets, Christine's tailored program is not a diet at all, but a revolution in the way we think about the foods we eat. *Skinny Chicks* is required reading for all my patients."

—Marc Mani, MD, FACS, board-certified plastic surgeon

SKINNY CHICKS DON'T EAT SALADS

STOP STARVING, START EATING. . .AND LOSING!

CHRISTINE AVANTI, CN

WITH SHARYN KOLBERG

RODALE

Rodale books may be purchased for business or promotional use or for special sales. For information, please write to: Special Markets Department, Rodale Inc., 733 Third Avenue, New York, NY 10017

Printed in the United States of America

Rodale Inc. makes every effort to use acid-free ∞, recycled paper ♻.

Book design by Susan Eugster

Library of Congress Cataloging-in-Publication Data

Avanti, Christine.
    Skinny chicks don't eat salads : stop starving, start eating . . . and losing / Christine Avanti.
       p.   cm.
    Includes bibliographical references.
    ISBN-13 978–1–60529–997–6 hardcover
    ISBN-13 978–1–60529–478–0 paperback
    1. Reducing diets.   2. Women—Health and hygiene.   I. Title.
RM222.2.A928 2009
613.2'5—dc22   2009001982

Distributed to the trade by Macmillan

2 4 6 8 10 9 7 5 3 1 paperback

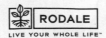

We inspire and enable people to improve their lives and the world around them

For more of our products visit **rodalestore.com** or call 800-848-4735

To all women who have

struggled needlessly to lose weight.

May you find peace and revelation

as you go on this journey, just like I did.

Contents

Introduction

Are you one of those people whose idea of dieting is starving yourself all day—and then stuffing yourself with a great big salad at night? Have you tried this approach and been happy with the results? Of course not. Because without ever having met you, I know that even if you lost weight in the short term, you gained it all back. We just can't live on salad alone.

I know, because I've been there myself. The Skinny Chicks program came out of my own need to get off the diet merry-go-round, to get fit and healthy and stop making myself crazy with food. I lived the life of eating salads during the day and bingeing on sweets at night. I guinea-pigged my way through every diet gimmick there was. I cycled through all the major diets: the Atkins diet, the grapefruit diet, the cabbage soup diet, the Mayo Clinic diet, the Sugar Busters diet, to name a few. I tried over-the-counter supplements and diet aids, Chinese herbs, and, at one point during my twenties, I even stooped to stealing my grandfather's prescription Lasix (a diuretic) to lose weight. When that didn't work, I paid someone to hypnotize me so I could get my eating under control. Needless to say, that didn't work either—and I was out $100. I didn't know or care whether I lost water weight, muscle tissue, or fat. I only cared about making the numbers on the scale go down.

After I had exhausted every possible fad diet and weight loss trick, I finally gave up and looked up. I prayed for God to point me in the proper direction. Then I met a nutritionist who suggested I learn more about food and the body if I really wanted to understand how to lose weight. As many of my clients do today, I argued with my nutritionist. I was very emotional about food, and I wanted to cling to my habits. I basically wanted her seal of approval for my existing ways. It took a lot of persuasion for me to let go of the low-carb concept. But eventually I realized that even though my background was in modeling, fitness, and personal training, I didn't fundamentally understand what was preventing me from losing weight. I decided to get certified as a nutritionist, and there I found the answer to my prayers.

I learned that eating too little food would slow down my metabolism more and more; that eating too much would cause fat storage; and finally that eating to keep blood sugar levels stable was the key to avoiding sugar cravings and thus gaining the weight back.

It was difficult for me to accept these concepts. All I wanted to do was restrict carbs and calories and watch the scale magically drop 10 pounds in a week, as it had so many times before.

But somehow, it all finally clicked. I started to eat balanced meals such as low-fat cottage cheese mixed with fresh fruit and yogurt, topped with crunchy walnuts; banana–peanut butter smoothies; and pumpkin pancakes (all of these recipes are in this book), and I went from a size 12 to a size 5 in 3 months. Best of all I was eating real food, not diet food, and those insatiable cravings for sweets and salty carbs were virtually eliminated. I was so excited to be "freed" from the bondage of "dieting" that I vowed to get this message to all the people who were suffering just like me. It was one of the best things that ever happened to me.

By eating the Skinny Chicks way, you *will* lose weight—anywhere from 2 to 8 pounds in the first 2 weeks alone—and you'll notice an improvement in your moods and overall outlook on life as well.

What's so great about this weight loss plan is that it is not a diet—it is an *eating plan.* I will teach you some basic body science principles regarding weight loss that will resonate with you the moment you read them. On my eating plan, you will learn how to program your metabolism to burn fat and save muscle 24 hours a day. Most people on this plan first notice weight loss in their midsection; then they notice an increase in energy and a happier mood, usually within the first week. Even better, you will not feel deprived or undernourished. You will never starve yourself because you'll be eating four or even five fully balanced meals a day (that's right, I said four or five meals a day, not three meals and two snacks). In fact, you might be tempted to say, as did one Skinny Chick client of mine, "Are you sure this isn't a gain-weight program?" I promised her, and I promise you, it's not.

The Skinny Chicks program is for people who have real lives and live in the real world, with jobs, families, and other responsibilities. My nutrition plan works for today's fast-paced lifestyle. I've included fast-food meals, upscale restaurant meals, and delicious, healthy recipes you can cook for yourself and your family. I've also included more than 60 quick "grab and go" meals—great for college students and busy working moms alike.

You're going to eat normal meals. You don't cut out carbs, you don't cut out fats, you don't cut out sugar. You can have desserts. You won't be eating boiled chicken and steamed broccoli at every meal. And best of all, you won't be eating salads for dinner.

The Skinny Chicks plan is the healthiest way to lose weight and keep it off. You don't have to starve yourself (in fact, you'll be defeating your dieting goals if you do). You don't have to weigh and measure your food. You don't have to cut out carbs. You don't have to be perfect. You can have pasta. You can even have sweets and chips (I'll tell you which ones are best and how and when to eat them). You can exercise a moderate amount and get the benefits you need. If you want to eat a salad, be my guest—I'll tell you how to make it right. In other words, you can live in the real world and still lose weight. I know, because that's the life I live. And I love it.

My goal is to explain it to you so that it's easy, so that it makes sense, and so that you'll really understand how the food you eat will affect your body and your life. I'm going to lay it out in a way that will change the way you eat forever.

So put down the salad fork and get ready to enjoy eating again. Before you know it, you'll be a Skinny Chick just like the hundreds and hundreds of clients I've helped with my Skinny Chicks program. You have nothing to lose but your cravings!

PART I

SKINNY CHICKS

LEARN THE

SCIENCE

CHAPTER 1

How Salads Got Us into Big Fat Trouble

4:00 on a Tuesday morning

I roll my puffy body off the edge of my warm, fluffy pillow-top bed. I'm suffering from a "food hangover." Why? Because last night, while discussing the ex-boyfriend with my beloved Aunt Sandra, I munched through an entire box of Ritz crackers, a jar of marshmallow cream, and a jar of Skippy peanut butter. Now I'm bloated from all that sodium and feel like a huge brick is sitting in my lower stomach.

So I do what I do every morning: gulp down two pots of coffee. Not two cups, two *pots*. That's why I need to wake up so very early; I need enough time to drink the coffee and visit the bathroom several times before heading to the gym to teach my hour-long Spinning class. Of course, I skip breakfast—I have to make up for all the calories consumed during last night's cracker–peanut butter–marshmallow sandwich binge.

I go to the gym and teach my Spin class, and work out as hard as I can.

8:30 a.m.

After class I'm famished and shaking because my blood sugar is so low. I'm so mad about bingeing last night, though, that I decide to skip breakfast, resist my hunger, and head home to take a shower. Afterward, I go down into the kitchen to prepare the lunch I'll take to the office: a BIG salad. It's gotta be BIG because I'm starving like an abandoned alley kitten and I still have hours to go before lunchtime, so I use a whole head of iceberg lettuce, a bell pepper, half of a cucumber, three stalks of celery, one large beefsteak tomato, one broccoli crown, one cauliflower crown, artichoke hearts (canned in water, not oil, of course), sprouts, and a half a bottle of low-cal ranch dressing.

1:00 p.m.

Nine hours after waking up, I'm finally ready to eat my first meal. At this point, I am really forgetful, agitated, and feeling so shaky I can barely remember my own name. I am so excited to take my first bite, because (a) it's healthier than what I ate last night and (b) I'm finally on the right track with my eating! Now I'm sure to lose weight.

3:00 p.m.

I'm still full from my lunch salad and I feel pretty good. And yet . . . I feel like I *need* to have something sweet. I find myself fantasizing about a chocolate chip cookie; don't I deserve at *least* one? After all, I've been awake since 4:00 a.m., I worked out like a banshee, and the only thing I've eaten all day is a salad! How much damage can one cookie do? I'm going for that cookie and then—I promise—I will get back on track.

3:30 p.m.

At the deli, my special chocolate chip cookie is warm, soft, moist, and smells like fresh-baked heaven. I love it. I *need* it. Hey—it's gone already! That wasn't even close to enough. I buy a mini lemon cake (it's made with fruit, right? It must be healthy) and as I devour it, the battle inside my head begins:

Christine . . . what the $%#@ are you doing? This is not on your diet.
You're such a loser, you can't even resist sweets for less than 24 hours.
Your diet is shot.
So what? Fine. I'm a loser. Who cares!

I buy two more mini lemon cakes and four more chocolate chip cook-ies and sneak them back to the office in my handbag. I eat them all within 2 hours, keeping the door to my office—where I work as the aer-obics manager of a popular LA health club—closed.

10:00 p.m.

I decided not to eat dinner because I had so many calories during my afternoon diet meltdown. Around 10:00 p.m., I have a small serving of nonfat frozen yogurt, figuring that that must be okay since I haven't had dinner. I decide I can have a second serving because the first one was so small, and this time I add some caramel syrup. (The caramel syrup bottle reads "fat free," after all.) The rest of the evening continues with more sweets, and I honestly can't stop myself. More than I crave love, companionship, or any emotional need—I crave sugar. The more I eat, the more I crave. These are not subtle cravings; they rule my every thought as well as my actions. Sugar is my significant other—like a toxic boyfriend that I can't break up with.

As I down these treats, I carry on a running argument with myself: *Am I a sugar addict? How can I be, when I'm so good that I exercise, skip meals, and eat only salad?* I want to sleep, but I'm so wired from all the sugar that I can't turn off the voices in my head.

I am completely out of control.

What I didn't realize was that I craved sugar because I basically fasted for the first 9 hours of my day. I had convinced myself that if I skipped break-fast, ate a BIG salad for lunch, skipped dinner, and ate "just a few" sweets during the day, I would finally lose weight. I kept this up for several years. It may have been a twisted way of thinking, but it was my reality.

And that is how salads got me into big fat trouble. I believe this is how salads get lots of girls into big fat trouble. Guys don't do this . . . it's only girls who eat this way and convince ourselves that it's "low-calorie eating." When we see slim women eating "real" food, we think to our-selves, "Oh, she has a special blessing from God, and that's why she can

Skinny Chick 10-Week Transformation

NAME: JULIA S.

AGE: 34

TOTAL POUNDS LOST: 27.25

TOTAL INCHES LOST: 31.5

I started gaining weight about 4 years ago, and each year it seemed like I gained more than the year before. This was a big change for me. As a child, I was very active. I played a lot of sports, and I never had a problem with food. My family is very health conscious. We all work out and eat well. So I could not figure out why I was gaining this weight.

Part of it was definitely my social lifestyle. I was drinking and partying and hanging out late at night, and I got a little carried away. I wasn't organizing my time properly. When partying and eating and drinking became a priority, I knew I had to back off.

Christine helped me change some bad habits. I now have breakfast every day, something I never did before. I learned to combine proteins with carbs. And, of course, I learned that skinny girls don't eat salads. I used to say, "I'm watching my weight, I'll just eat a salad." I realize that doesn't work. But if I have a nice *healthy* salad, with a little chicken or some egg white, I feel better and can stick to my goals. I've learned to enjoy foods that are healthy. Double bacon cheeseburgers are great, but they're not giving my body the nutrition it needs.

Life can be so overwhelming, and sometimes it feels you're just living day to day, trying to make it, not really achieving the things you set out to do. Now, with the Skinny Chicks program, I know that once I put my mind to doing something, I can do it. I feel inspired to let the real Julia come out and shine. I look back and see that all my fat was covering so much beauty. Can I just pat myself on the back?

eat normal meals and I'm stuck with eating rabbit food." Let me be the first to tell you that you *can* eat "normal" food and be thin, too. It all starts with stepping away from the salad mentality and learning the truth about what makes us crave what we shouldn't eat and why eating what we shouldn't is so bad for us.

Why Skinny Chicks Don't Eat Salads

Back in 1999, I was 30 pounds overweight, and it seemed like nothing could help me lose the extra pounds. Now, after learning about how food works in the body, I am in the best shape of my life. I've come to realize that weight loss is not accomplished through a fad diet or TV exercise gimmick; it is a matter first and foremost of the heart. Once your heart is onboard, it is a matter of educating yourself about sensible nutrition.

One day, two friends and I were dining at a popular LA eatery. Deep in conversation, I didn't take time to study the menu carefully, and when the waiter asked for my order, I just went with a salad. As is often the case, my two girlfriends echoed my order, assuming that I—a nutritionist—had made a healthy choice. When our meals arrived, all three of us looked at the salads and back at each other . . . and burst out laughing. They looked like erupting volcanoes, massive piles of breaded chicken strips and chunks of three different kinds of cheese, all smothered in a creamy dressing.

We were embarrassed by the sheer quantity of food in front of us. The salads were not only unhealthy, they were definitely *not* conducive to losing weight. In fact, these "healthy" dishes probably contained more than 1,000 calories! I told my friends that anybody "dieting" on these salads would become obese within weeks, and then blurted out, "I'll tell you one thing . . . skinny chicks don't eat salads!"

We think of salads as a very light meal (as opposed to a big steak or a plate of lasagna), and indeed, half a head of iceberg lettuce contains only about 39 calories, with trace amounts of vitamins and no fat. No wonder most people believe that eating salad is a healthy alternative to high-calorie foods and a basic building block of any weight loss plan.

But when it comes to nutrition and weight loss, all salads are not created equal. For our grandparents, a salad usually consisted of lettuce, tomatoes, and cucumbers, drizzled with a bit of vinegar and olive oil. Have you watched a cooking show lately? Or eaten in a restaurant? Everything comes super-sized with a list of ingredients that takes up half the menu page.

Nowadays, when you order a salad from any restaurant, be it a fast-food spot or an upscale eatery, you are going to get a huge amount of lettuce topped with two or three kinds of cheese, candied pecans or slivered almonds, breaded and fried chicken, bacon bits or dried cranberries, and fried tortilla strips or buttery fried croutons—all drenched with calorie-laden dressing.

After the volcano salad incident, I decided to do a little field research. I ordered salads from several popular restaurants and had them pack every ingredient separately. I weighed all the individual toppings, plugged them into my food database, and added up the calories in each salad. What I found out was that there were actually more calories in a Cobb salad than a frosting-smothered Cinnabon! The results were so unbelievable—shocking in fact—that *E! News* did a story on them.

SALADS	CALORIES	FAT (G)	CARB (G)	PROTEIN (G)
Cheesecake Factory Caesar Salad	1,699	145	44	65
Applebee's Stacked Tostada Salad	1,409	119	38	50
Cheesecake Factory Cobb Salad	1,340	96	47	74
Applebee's Oriental Chicken Salad	1,237	74	91	58
Chili's Southwestern Cobb Salad	1,117	82	40	56
Macaroni Grill Chicken Caesar Salad	675	44	14	50

In contrast, here are some fast foods that we would never dare touch while dieting, yet actually contain fewer calories than the typical restaurant salad.

FAST FOODS	CALORIES	FAT (G)	CARB (G)	PROTEIN (G)
Burger King Whopper	678	37	53	31
In-N-Out Double Double with Cheese	670	41	40	37
McDonald's Big Mac with Cheese	563	32	43	25
Dairy Queen Double Homestyle Cheeseburger	540	31	30	35
Taco Bell Seven Layer Burrito	530	22	67	18
Wendy's Double Cheeseburger	458	25	34	25
Taco Bell Double Decker Supreme	380	18	40	15

Of course, a small salad with a little bit of dressing before or after a meal is just fine. But substituting a salad for a more diverse variety of healthy and satisfying foods, and then chowing down on sugary treats as a reward for that "sacrifice," causes erratic blood sugar levels—just the opposite of what we need to lose weight.

The Key to Losing Weight

Before we go on, I'd like you to take a short quiz. Which of these symptoms have you experienced in the past 2 weeks?

- Headaches
- Sugar cravings
- Caffeine cravings
- Shakiness/dizziness
- Mood swings/irritability
- Lethargy/lack of energy
- Lack of concentration
- Extreme hunger

Skinny Chick 10-Week Transformation

NAME: JESSICA C.

AGE: 29

TOTAL POUNDS LOST: 27

TOTAL INCHES LOST: 27.5

I've been overweight since about first grade. I was a latchkey kid growing up, and I didn't have much adult supervision in the morning or afternoon. When I got home from school, I did what kids normally do: eat junk food and watch TV. I lived on instant noodles, peanut butter, and Doritos. When you're a kid, you don't know any better; you just go with what tastes good. Then I went to college and the problem got even worse because I had free rein with junk food.

When I was 20 years old, my mother's sister passed away from complications of obesity. She was only 50 years old. She was diabetic and had had a lot of health issues that come from being overweight. That was a wake-up call for me, and it made me take a look at my life. I began to eat better and make better choices, and I tried to exercise more. It helped a lot. I went from a size 24 to about a size 18. For somebody who weighed about 250 pounds, that was a big difference. But then I stopped losing weight.

I tried a lot of different diets, none of which really worked. I tried the Zone diet, just not eating, and even a crazy diet that was supposed to take off 10 pounds in 3 days. No surprise, it didn't work. After those 3 days, you lose about 5 pounds, but you're so demoralized and hungry that you gain about 7 pounds back. All the diets I tried were too hard to follow, and they didn't really let you live your life.

And *all* of these diets tell you to have meals made of salads. To make your salad have more pizzazz, you keep throwing vegetables in there. You start to hate vegetables, which makes it even worse. At the end of the day, you eat the same thing every day and you just hate it all.

A year and a half ago I got engaged, and ever since then I've been even more focused on losing weight. Each time I start a new diet, I stick with it for about a month and then life gets in the way. Now that I'm planning a wedding, I have a lot to do and no time for diets that require a lot of cooking, a lot of different ingredients, or just a lot of sacrifice.

And then the Skinny Chicks program came along. It allowed me to live my life—and I've now lost 27 pounds and gone down several sizes.

Even if I weren't getting married, I would love this program because it's a life change, not just a temporary thing. It's easy to follow. It doesn't require any cooking skills, no secret formula, no counting points. It's flexible, too. It's easy to estimate your portions so you don't have to weigh and measure everything. You just listen to your body. If you're really hungry, then you may have a little bit more. It's not rocket science.

This is a way of life I can continue to follow. What greater gift than to know you can have good health forever? It doesn't get much better than that.

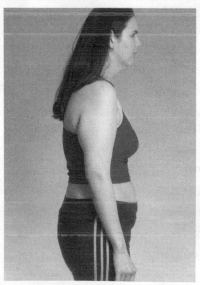 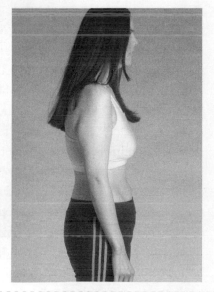

If you checked off several items on the list, you are riding the blood sugar roller coaster, a cycle that will have you feeling cheerful one minute and down in the dumps the next . . . not to mention overtired, overwhelmed, and overweight.

What if I were to tell you that keeping your blood sugar on a healthy, even keel would help you get rid of these annoying and debilitating symptoms without starvation or deprivation—and help you lose weight in the process? All you have to do is make a few simple, non-extreme dietary changes.

If you do occasionally experience the symptoms above, don't hit the panic button. It just means you haven't eaten for a while and your brain cells need a little fuel. Where do they get that fuel? From the carbohydrates you eat (so much for the "healthy" no-carb diet).

In this book, I'll explain the basics of blood sugar, what it does in your body, and why keeping blood sugar levels stable is the single most important concept in losing weight. It also increases your energy and has a host of other benefits. So, if you take away just one principle from this book, let it be this: *The key to losing weight and keeping it off is keeping your blood sugar stable.* Understand this concept, apply it to how and what you eat, and it will be transformative.

What Is Blood Sugar, Anyway?

Blood sugar (glucose) is by no means a bad thing. In fact, our bodies need glucose to function; it's the primary fuel that our cells use. Some cells, such as brain, nerve, and red blood cells, can run only on glucose. Your blood sugar level refers to the amount of glucose in your blood.

As I said before, glucose comes from the carbohydrates we eat. When most people think of carbs, they automatically think of french fries, white bread, rice, pasta, and sweets like cakes and doughnuts. But veggies, whole grains, fruits, and beans are also packed with carbs—and in fact, they're the best sources of carbs. Here's another important factoid to remember: Whether the carbs you eat come from pasta, rice, or grains, no matter how much you eat at one sitting, your brain cells will need more carbs 4 hours later. The brain and nervous system don't store glucose. When glucose levels are low, the body begins to break down liver and muscle glycogen (glucose) for fuel. So, no new carbs, no fresh fuel for brain cells, and the body begins to break down its own tissues—thus the headache you get when you eat a late lunch. Carbs get a bad rap. A billion-dollar industry has sprung up around the notion that carbs are evil. (Witness the shelves at your grocery store; they're stocked with no-carb and low-carb products.) How can something your body needs to function, to run its own command center—your brain—be bad for you? Simply put, they're not. As a nutritionist, I get into a lot of confrontations with bright people who are convinced they need to cut out carbs to lose weight. The reality is that you *need* carbs every 4 hours. But the trick is getting the right amount of the right carbs at the right times. In this book, you'll learn how many carbs you really need to eat, what you need to eat them with, and the best times to eat them. And, as you'll find out, it's as easy as ABC.

In the next chapters, I'll explain the principles behind the Skinny Chicks program and why it will work for you. You'll hear from real people how this program works in the real world through testimonials from some of my private practice clients as well as from some participants in the Skinny Chicks test group. When I started to write this book, I wanted to be sure that the program I developed would be just as effective as the individualized plans I create for my private clients, so I invited a group of people to go on the Skinny Chicks journey with me. Twenty intrepid women followed the program in this book for 10 weeks, kept journals, and answered weekly questionnaires. The group lost a combined total of 310 pounds, an average of 15.5 pounds per person, 23 inches per person, and a total of 452 inches lost over 10 weeks! It was more successful than even I imagined. You'll meet some of these people throughout the book and hear their stories.

One important thing that came out of this group is that the Skinny Chicks program is redefining skinny. It's no longer the rail-thin, "I only eat lettuce" model. If a size 12 is skinny for you, that's great. For someone else, it might be a size 4. You're skinny when you're empowered with knowledge, when your blood sugar is balanced, and when you live a healthy lifestyle.

CHAPTER 2

The ABCs
of Weight Loss

Nutrition isn't simple. As with so many things in life, moderation is the key. If you take any nutritional solution too far, it doesn't work. The perfect example is eating zero carbs. Yes, you will lose weight because the body will eventually break down body fat for energy. There are only a couple of snafus: (1) it may promote the development of kidney stones, cause acidosis (increase the acidity of the body's fluids), decrease calcium balance, and increase the risk for bone loss; and (2) most of us will end up crawling into the kitchen in the middle of the night to get our hands on the stuff our brains need: cakes, cookies, doughnuts, ice cream, anything with carbs in it. This is no way to live a happy life. Here's the thing: You don't have to give up carbs to live a happy life. You don't have to become a "slave to the crave" that hits you when your blood sugar is out of whack.

Your blood sugar starts out on the low side in the morning because while you sleep, you essentially fast for 7 to 8 hours or more. Your Skinny Chicks goal is to keep your blood sugar stabilized, which is defined as anywhere between 80 and 120 milligrams of glucose per deciliter of blood. Anywhere above or below this range can result in fat storage, as indicated by the unhappy faces in the chart on page 15.

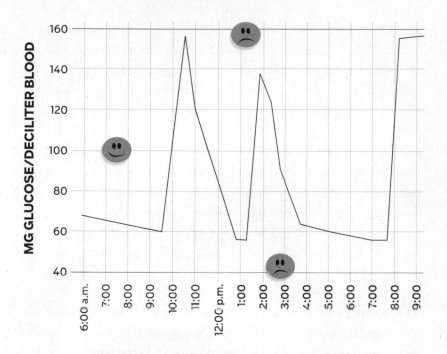

ERRATIC BLOOD SUGAR

If you are like me, you are a busy woman and you don't always have time to eat breakfast. Most of us consider that to be a good thing because we actually think that starving ourselves is the way to lose weight. But take a look at the chart above and check out what happens to blood sugar levels on a typical day for a typical salad eater.

Now, remember that brain cells can only function with glucose for fuel, and since the body doesn't store it in a readily accessible state, you need to give it more approximately every 4 hours. This applies to every human being alive. When you wake up in the morning and you haven't eaten for 8 hours or more, your body has already dipped into your reserve fuel storage (glycogen from your liver and muscle tissues—more on that later) and the tank is empty.

When we break down and succumb to that morning Frappuccino, our blood sugar shoots from super low to super high. Hunger goes away but returns quickly as blood sugar rapidly drops, leaving us hungrier than ever for "real food." Once we finally eat our big salad, we have a little—

but not nearly enough—of what our body needs: carbs. Throughout the rest of the day, we are essentially miserable and on a constant lookout for a little treat. Remember, the brain has barely had its required glucose all day. At night, the need for fuel is stronger than our willpower could ever be, so we cave in and eat sweets like Miss Piggy on a breakup binge.

What happens when you drink that Frappuccino or eat a bunch of sweets on an empty stomach? Your body gets flooded with glucose, which causes your pancreas to release large amounts of insulin to carry the glucose to the cells for fuel. This puts us in a hyperglycemic (spiked blood sugar) state, and if there is more glucose than our cells can use, the extra calories are stored as fat. Insulin does the job of clearing away blood glucose extremely well, and soon blood sugar levels are low again. That's when you find yourself feeling hungry again an hour or two later.

The Insulin/Blood Sugar Connection

As you can see from the chart on page 15, your blood sugar levels are influenced by what you eat and when you eat it. You've probably heard of insulin and blood sugar levels before, but you may have thought they were only important to people with diabetes. Actually, we should all be concerned about blood sugar, especially those of us who are trying to lose weight—meaning most Americans.

The easiest way to understand the way the glucose/insulin process works is to think of insulin as a package delivery system. I like to call it FatEx. Inside the FatEx truck are packages of glucose. The truck travels around in the interstitial fluid of the body (the fluid that is found in between cells), pulls up to a cell, knocks on the door, and says, "Hi, I'm here to deliver a package." The cell door opens up, accepts the package, and gets its glucose delivery. The FatEx truck then continues on its route and travels around to the next cell. Sometimes the cell door doesn't open; the response is, "Oh no, we don't need a package of glucose right now, we have enough. Go to a different cell." So the little FatEx truck keeps on driving around to all the cells, and eventually the cells become "insulin resistant" and stop accepting glucose.

When that happens, the insulin FatEx truck is forced to circulate around in the bloodstream and in between cells until finally the body says, "Enough. We don't have room for any more packages." What does anyone do when they run out of room? They put the leftovers in storage units. The body's storage space is the fat cell. At this point, the conversion of glucose to fatty acids is accomplished by insulin's activation of several enzymes, especially one called lipoprotein lipase. When that happens, the FatEx truck leaves a special rush delivery on your rear end and parks itself on your hips!

The point is that although you need carbs every 4 hours, you don't want to flood your system with glucose by eating too many carbs at one time. But you also don't want to deprive your system of glucose by eating too *few* carbs.

Let's take a look at a stable blood sugar chart below. Here we have a balanced meal that includes protein, carbs, and healthy fats, eaten within 1 hour of waking up. This is followed by another small, balanced meal every 4 hours throughout the day. The result? Blood sugar levels that are

STABILIZED BLOOD SUGAR

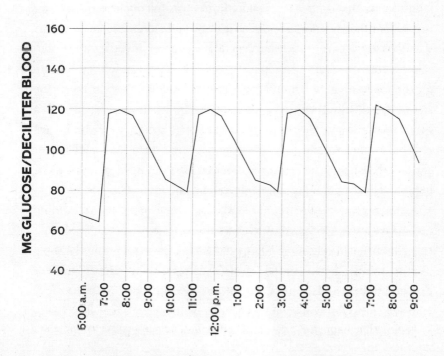

never too high and never too low. This is the optimal condition for fat burning because your body draws energy from blood sugar (from food) and fat storage. What's more, you have steady energy and stable hormones (more on these in Chapter 3) *and* you aren't starving to death.

As Easy as A, B, C, and D

Understanding blood sugar, hormonal responses, fat storage, and fat burning in your body is one thing, but actually making it work in your real life so that you can lose weight is another thing entirely. That is why I break it down into ABC & D: Amount, Balance, Clock, and Darnit, Get Your Lazy Butt on the Treadmill. Each of these is explained in detail in subsequent chapters, but here they are in a nutshell.

Amount: Many people think that dieting means eating less. But the truth is, slashing calories alone will not help you lose weight. Let me explain. When you skip breakfast or any other meal, you slow your resting metabolic rate—the number of calories your body burns at rest. Metabolism is the process whereby the body converts food into energy, uses it for repairs, or stores it as fat for future use. In simple terms, a faster metabolism burns calories more efficiently and stores less fat. A slower metabolism burns calories less efficiently and therefore causes more calories to be stored as fat. When insufficient food is present in the stomach, ghrelin levels are high (ghrelin is a hormone, produced by cells lining the stomach, that stimulates the appetite). Ghrelin levels increase prior to a meal and decrease after a meal. If you don't eat enough, your ghrelin levels will keep poking at your insides, saying, "Feed me! Feed me!" Chapter 3 will explain how to determine how much food you need to satisfy these ghrelin gremlins, lose (or maintain) weight, and stay healthy.

Balance: Eating to keep your blood sugar stable is not about starving; just the opposite. On the Skinny Chicks' eating plan you can have it all. In fact, the key to success is having it *all at once* by combining the three leading macronutrients found in the foods you eat: proteins, high-fiber carbs, and healthy fats. If you want to give your body optimum fuel while burning fat, you've got to balance your blood sugar levels. Too high or too low and you're storing fat or losing muscle tissue. I'll tell you exactly what you need to eat—and when—in order to stabilize your blood sugar, save muscle, and, most importantly, burn fat. When you read Chapter 4, you will learn a diet principle so easy and so logical, you will wonder why you never knew it before. And when you put it into practice, you will wish you had known it a long time ago.

Keeping balance in the body is vitally important. Think about what happens when you drink wine on an empty stomach. It goes "straight to your head." It is absorbed into your bloodstream very quickly and delivered directly to your brain. However, if you eat something along with the wine, it slows down the delivery to the brain. The same thing happens when you sit down at a restaurant, ravenously hungry, and start eating bread before dinner. Bread on an empty stomach is absorbed into the bloodstream very quickly, causing your blood sugar level to spike. The trick in Chapter 4 will help you slow down this process and sustain your energy throughout the day.

Clock: The symptoms listed in the quiz in Chapter 1 most often appear when you've waited too long between meals. The Skinny Chicks program recommends that you eat every 4 hours. That's because your brain and nervous system can store only enough glucose to fuel them for about 4 hours. After that, they go for the stored glycogen (the main form in which glucose is stored in the body) in your liver and muscle tissue. And when you break down liver and muscle tissue, *you dramatically slow down metabolism.* In simple terms, if you go too long without food, your body thinks there is a food shortage and your metabolism tends to slow down. Meals eaten too far apart promote fat storage, low energy, headaches, and sugar cravings.

Darnit, Get Your Lazy Butt on the Treadmill: We all lose muscle mass as we get older. We can also lose muscle mass from lack of use. Muscle cells are about eight times more metabolically demanding than fat cells, so the greater your proportion of muscle to fat, the faster your metabolic rate will be.

Eating decent-size meals every 4 hours was a dream come true for a body image–obsessed girl like me. And eating delicious meals such as a Denver omelet (eggs, Canadian bacon, peppers, and onions) with toast; pasta with meat sauce; grilled chicken breast sandwiches; or cheese with fruit and wine? That doesn't sound like diet food because it's *not*. The Skinny Chicks plan isn't about depriving and starving; it's about giving your body what it really needs, when it needs it.

DON'T IGNORE YOUR ABCS

The silliest thing is that the ABCs are all naturally built into every human being—we just ignore them. If you are a parent, you know that a newborn baby needs food every few hours. Toddlers are constantly hungry and ask for food when they need it. They don't care if it's "time" for a meal or not; they just know their bodies need fuel. Adults learn to ignore hunger pangs if they're in the middle of an important work project, only to overeat several hours later when they finally get a chance to take a break. When they follow that pattern week after week, month after month, year after year, they end up in my office complaining that they are fat even though they eat healthfully. Surprisingly, most clients come to me with the same story. It goes something like this: "In my high school and college years I could eat whatever I wanted and never gained weight, but now I just have to look at food and I put on the pounds." Then they blame it on their age. But the truth is, they are gaining weight now because all those days of skipping meals have caused their metabolisms to slow to a crawl—so that their bodies cling to every calorie they *do* eat.

Meet Giuliana, Who Woke Up Rundown

Giuliana Rancic was on top of the world. She had met the love of her life and landed her dream job as the host of *E! News* on the E! Network. Life was good! So why did she feel so awful? She was exhausted all the time. She had absolutely no energy and was downright cranky. Plus, she had put on about 10 pounds. That might not seem like much, but for a girl as small as Giuliana, the extra weight added up to her not being able to fit into her clothes. (Not to mention that every day, her weight gain was reflected back to her plus 10 pounds on television.)

Instead of waking up in the morning filled with excitement and antici-
pation, she woke up feeling sad and rundown. She didn't know it at the
time, but her weariness and malaise were the result of her unhealthy
eating habits. Here is her story.

*Most days I was so busy at work that I didn't make time to eat. On a
typical day I would skip breakfast and lunch. By dinnertime I was so
famished I would eat not one, but two dinners—I had to make up for the
meals I skipped during the day, didn't I? I would hardly finish stuffing
myself before my sweet tooth started calling. Why shouldn't I have a bowl of
frozen yogurt, or a carton even? I had hardly eaten all day. The morning
after a sugar binge, I would wake up feeling like I had a hangover. Not to
mention the emotional hangover—I was so full of shame and so angry at
myself that I'd swear off food for the whole day only to repeat the cycle at
night when I got home.*

*I bought every diet book on the market; I spent hours on the Internet
searching for advice, but nothing helped. I was depressed and at my wit's end.
That's when I turned to Christine for help. The first time I met with Christine, she explained to me that my eating habits were causing blood sugar
levels to spike then dip. She clued me in to the fact that the way I was eating
was causing my uncontrollable sugar cravings and that my blood sugar ups
and downs were actually the reason for my weight gain and my inability to
drop the pounds. Right then and there, I signed up for her program, and I
haven't turned back. At first I thought it was willpower that was behind my
ability to put the brakes on my nightly sugar binges, then I realized the reality
was that I hadn't conquered my cravings, I had stopped having them!
Christine's program enabled me to lose the weight, but even more importantly, I now wake up in the morning feeling excited about my day.*

There's No Need to Be Hungry

Like Giuliana, many of us are confused by all the diet info out there,
and this lack of knowledge can severely affect our quality of life, for a
lifetime! We try this diet and that, but ultimately we go back to our old

Skinny Chick 10-Week Transformation

NAME: RUTH W.

AGE: 39

TOTAL POUNDS LOST: 15

TOTAL INCHES LOST: 18.5

I was pretty lean as a child and up to the age of about 24. After my first child, I lost all the baby fat. But after the second, I didn't. I just kept gaining weight. I didn't really notice that I was gaining weight until my husband started to notice. He still loves me, but it affected our relationship. I tried diet pills; I tried exercise. Nothing was working. I never imagined that eating more could actually help me lose weight. I was skeptical. I thought, Is this a get-fat plan? But this morning my husband said, "I want to thank Christine because you look hot!"

I learned that it is very important to look at the labels on everything you buy. I've reduced the amount of fat in my diet. I'm Latin, and I've learned how to cook fat-free Mexican food. I learned how to cook a lot of things that are low-calorie, homemade. I stopped eating out so much. I cook for a few hours on Sunday night after the baby is asleep. During the week, I can make 10 meals out of the chicken or fish I made on Sunday. It's inspired me to cook healthy meals for my whole family. My husband is actually losing weight on the program too.

I'm definitely continuing with the program. This program changed the way that I eat. It's really improved my life. It's changed my health, the way I feel about myself. I love that I can eat. I love that I look great. I love that I am healthier. I just can't believe what this program has done for me, for my body, for my health. It made me feel sexy again. It's changed my relationship with my husband. My husband is so grateful, and so am I.

bellwether of weight loss success (or so we think): hunger. Nobody wants to feel hungry, but many of us girls do for some portion of each day. Most people on a diet see hunger as an accomplishment; it must be doing some good because it feels so bad. I know that's how I felt, and it's how many of my clients feel when they first come to my office. You don't have to feel that way anymore. You can and should feel like a healthy, stable, empowered person who is capable of doing anything— not like someone who is weak, distracted by hunger, and miserable.

CHAPTER 3

It's the Amount That Counts

When it comes to nutrition, health, and weight loss, one of the topics that really gets me fired up is the idea that starving yourself will help you lose weight. My philosophy is that in order to lose weight, we should not be eating *less*; just the opposite—we should be eating *more*. One of the most important messages of this book is that you should never starve yourself. Skipping meals is what leads to overeating, and that's not a good thing.

I never want you to skip meals. In fact, as you'll soon see, I want you to *add* meals to your day. This is great news for everyone who loves to eat (and who doesn't?). But how much food should you be eating? How important is it to eat a healthy, balanced meal? To this day, there are many people in the health and fitness industry who say that it doesn't matter what you eat or when, and all that matters is the number of calories. These CICO (Calories In Calories Out) theorists believe that human nutrition is as simple as eat-more-weigh-more and eat-less-weigh-less. If you subscribe to this logic, the plan of skipping meals and centering your diet around big fat salads looks like a winning strategy, right? And it would work fine if it weren't for one small glitch: human physiology.

"I'm Starving, but I'm Losing Weight"

Just for the sake of argument, let's see what happens if you actually avoid food for, say, 24 hours. Somewhere around 24 hours after your last meal, your body enters a state known as ketosis. (This state can also be reached by eating only protein and no carbs for approximately 24 to 48 hours.) In this state, your body begins to break down fat for fuel. If you are stranded on a deserted island and you have some extra body fat, this might help you last longer than your skinny sisters. But in the real world, you are bombarded with food temptation all day every day. By the 24th hour, you are insatiably thirsty, you have a bad taste in your mouth and the breath of a dragon, you have a nonstop headache, and you are moping around like a hound dog. But guess what? You will be burning fat.

Before you go and just stop eating, let's think about some other things. Your hair and skin will be getting no nutrients, so your face will start to look haggard and worn. Your hair requires protein; A, B, and D vitamins; iron; and a variety of other nutrients, so starving on and off for as little as 6 months is likely to make your hair brittle, frizzy, and damaged. It will take you an entire year to regrow healthy hair. I don't know about you, but that is pretty much enough to convince me that starvation is not the way to go.

A more important consideration is that your muscles—including the most important muscle, your heart—are being broken down for fuel. Your metabolism has been reduced to the slowest possible crawl; fat burning is minimized since you have nothing to "eat" besides your own body.

The body consists of trillions of cells, and all day long, each one performs its little cellular processes. Each of these processes requires various nutrients, enzymes, and compounds that come from the foods we eat. On a starvation diet, the cells just don't get what they need and bad things start to happen. Let's look at the implications listed in the chart on page 26.

As you can see, starvation is not the way to healthy weight loss. Even if you have an iron will, you are doing more harm to your body than good. If you are like most people, you will find that rather than fasting

BODY PART	WHAT HAPPENS	WHAT'S THE PROBLEM?
Bones	Weak bones, osteoporosis	Lack of calcium
Energy level	Anemia (tired all the time)	Lack of vitamin E, vitamin K, folate, iron, zinc, vitamin B_6, or vitamin B_{12}
Eyes	Dark circles under eyes	Not enough iron
Gastrointestinal tract	Constipation	Lack of fiber
Hair	Depigmentation (gray hair), slow hair growth	Not enough protein
Hair	Hair loss	Not enough biotin, B_6, B_{12}, or folate
Hair	Dry and brittle hair	Not enough iodine
Mouth	Bleeding gums	Not enough vitamin C
Mouth	Cracked lips; swollen, dark red tongue	Not enough vitamin B_2 (riboflavin)
Skin	Dry, scaly, old-looking skin	Not enough essential fatty acids, vitamin E, or protein
Skin	Greasy skin	Not enough vitamin B_2 (riboflavin)
Soft tissues	Delayed wound healing	Not enough vitamin A, vitamin C, or zinc

entirely, you are actually snacking throughout the day to feed your body's basic need for glucose, and then overeating at night.

Why does this happen? The answer is that your body uses regulatory and counter-regulatory hormones to balance the chemicals in your body. This is why we dieters get so nutty! Insulin, cortisol, epinephrine (adrenaline), ghrelin, and leptin all play a role. Remember those ghrelin gremlins that are poking at your stomach, begging to be fed? When people say, "she's hormonal," it's not just a phrase. Research studies have shown that the levels of these hormones in the bloodstream fluctuate greatly as a result of what we do—or don't—eat.

The "Okay, I'll Just Skip Breakfast" Myth

What about semi-starvation—just skipping a meal here or there? Let's see what happens then. Within 4 hours of any meal, your brain will once again be in need of fuel. The hormone ghrelin is released, causing hunger pangs. If you decide to "be good" and skip a meal, your brain isn't just going to shut off; it will turn to reserve storage, taking sugar in the form of glycogen from the muscle and liver tissues. As soon as the brain has to go to these tissues for fuel, it is going to do two things: (1) slow down your metabolism because it thinks you are starving; and (2) start aching. Most people think they are unique in getting a headache when they skip lunch. The reality is that all human beings get light-headed, headachy, and all the other symptoms of hypoglycemia when their blood sugar gets low.

Just as an illustration (the reality is a bit more complex), think of your body's fuel sources as reserve fuel tanks. We'll call them Tanks 1, 2, 3, and 4. Your body's Tank 1 is blood sugar energy from food. When you have recently eaten, your body is burning the least fat. When Tank 1 starts to get low (i.e., low blood sugar), your body dips into Tank 2—glycogen stored in the liver and muscle tissues—along with some body fat. Once Tank 2 runs out, your body starts to consume its own muscles and vital protein tissues and fat (Tank 3). After a day or more of starving (or no carbs), your body will go into ketosis and actively use a lot of fat—Tank 4—for energy.

The Skinny Chicks program keeps you going between Tank 1 and Tank 2. I want you to use Tank 2 because that is where the fat burning occurs, but I want you to avoid Tank 3 because it means a slowed metabolism and loss of muscle—not to mention hunger, hypoglycemia, and pain.

	BODY'S PRIMARY FUEL SOURCE	TIME ELAPSED SINCE LAST MEAL	ARE YOU BURNING FAT?	RESULTS
Tank 1	Blood sugar (glucose from carbs)	None (immediate)	Yes, if eating correctly	Energy from 50% blood sugar and 50% fat—speeds up metabolism for optimal fat burning
Tank 2	Glycogen (glucose) stored in liver and muscles	3 to 5 hours	Yes, if eating correctly	
Tank 3	Muscles and vital tissues	5 to 6 hours or more	Yes— but . . .	Dramatically slowed metabolism, consuming muscles
Tank 4	Body fat (ketosis)	24 to 72 hours	Yes— but . . .	Dramatically slowed metabolism, very damaging to body and metabolism

Let's not take this "slowed metabolism" thing lightly. Metabolism is commonly known as the breakdown of food inside the body and its transformation into energy. I define it as the sum of all the life processes of each of the trillions of cells in the body. With a faster metabolism, your body can burn more food, while a slower metabolism means that even when eating less, you can gain weight. When you eat the right amount at regular intervals, your body speeds up your metabolism. If your metabolism is faster, your body automatically burns fat all day and even at night when you are sleeping. When you starve yourself or skip a meal, your body thinks you're in a famine and it needs to help you survive. As Lawrence Cheskin, MD, of Johns Hopkins Weight Management Center in Baltimore describes it, " . . . when you're eating less for weight loss, your body begins to act as if it's being shortchanged. Your metabolism slows in an attempt to conserve fuel." It will slow everything down so that it does not burn as many calories, including your rate of digestion, your circulation, your breathing, and, of course, your brain and

Skinny Chick Chat

Dear Christine: I need to lose at least 20 pounds, and I've been eating one meal a day . . . if I can't lose weight on just one meal a day, how can I eat every 4 hours? You also mentioned that I would feel the symptoms of hypoglycemia if I don't eat every 4 hours, but I've been a one-meal-a-day person for years, and I never feel the symptoms of hypoglycemia. Can you tell me what is going on with my body?

SUZIE J., LOS ANGELES

Suzie: You're what I call a "body divorcée." Don't feel bad; I hear this in my office quite often. When you first began skipping meals and/or waiting too long between meals, your body tried to nudge at you via the symptoms of hypoglycemia. You say that you've been eating only one meal a day for a while, so you may not remember the subtle headaches, sugar cravings, depression, and lack of concentration. But I guarantee you felt at least one if not more of the symptoms of hypoglycemia when you first started skipping meals. The fact that you are not having those symptoms any longer is a sign of a severely damaged metabolism. Our relationships with our bodies can be compared with a marriage: In the beginning, the communication is very clear and blissful, but after several years of ignoring a nagging spouse, divorce (or at least estrangement) is the inevitable outcome. I believe our bodies are the same: Your body tried to notify you not to wait too long between meals by giving you the warning signs of hypoglycemia, but after years of trying to communicate with you, your body eventually gave up. Now you have zero communication and you don't feel the symptoms of hypoglycemia. But take heart. Your body is very resilient and forgiving. Once you begin eating every 4 hours on a regular schedule, your body will open communication with you again, and you will be on the road to regaining a healthy metabolism. Try it and see for yourself!

EAT WELL, CHRISTINE

nervous system functions. Then, when you have a late evening binge, your body can't burn the calories, and even small meals can result in fat storage. Metabolism is a hugely important concept in my program.

Common Pitfalls for Dieters

I hope I have now convinced you that you shouldn't *ever* starve yourself. But this is not a license to overeat at will. Overeating has become a huge problem in our country. The astonishing statistics say that 6 out of every 10 Americans are overweight; nearly 1 in 3 is obese. Since 1991, the obesity rate in adults has risen 60 percent. In North and South America, it is estimated that just under half of the region's children will be overweight by 2010, up from about 28 percent. Everyone is worried about weight, either their own or their loved one's. The subject of nutrition used to be the ultimate wet blanket of cocktail party conversation, but now I find that everybody wants to talk to me about it. Even people who are in pretty good shape are wondering how they gain weight so easily.

What happens when we eat too much? What if, for instance, you ate an entire German chocolate cake followed by a carrot cake chaser? (Unthinkable you say? Been there, done that. I ate entire cakes several times back in my salads and sweets days.) Even a less extreme example—say, following a large plate of pasta with an ice cream dessert—will trigger the same overeating effects. When you eat a huge helping of carbs, a ton of glucose is dumped into your bloodstream all at once, causing your blood sugar levels to skyrocket. In reaction to the inundation of glucose, a fleet of insulin FatEx trucks will be dispatched to deliver it. Only so much can be delivered to cells in need of fuel and to muscle and liver storage units; the rest will go into the one place that has an abundance of storage space: fat storage cells. This happens quickly (FatEx is very efficient), and before you know it, there is virtually no glucose left in your blood. It has literally gone from your lips to your hips. At that point, your blood sugar levels will take a nosedive—also not good. When levels fall too low, you get grouchy and hungry very quickly, even if you've eaten only 2 hours before. This is known as reactive hypoglycemia. Your brain tells you to reach for more food, sweet food. Sugar-free food will not do; the body needs real glucose. You're very likely to give in to this sweet craving and reach for a doughnut or a few chocolate chip cookies, which will cause the cycle to repeat itself.

Most of us are not eating an entire German chocolate cake at one sitting; more likely, it is a pastry from Starbucks on an empty stomach or a late night mini-binge of Ben & Jerry's. But either way, this overeating is causing a small amount of fat storage each time.

So why is it that we are so much heavier than we were even 10 years ago? There are many different pieces of the puzzle. Some people blame the obesity epidemic on our sedentary lifestyles of computers, TV, and video games. Sure, they are partially to blame. But to me, it's pure and simple: The reason is clearly our food intake. First of all, everything comes in an enormous portion size. Venti lattes, 64-ounce Big Gulps, super-sized meals, and restaurants serving on 15-inch dinner plates are all culprits. Another problem is the inescapable presence of so many new, delicious food creations consisting of highly refined carbs and fats. You pull up to a drive-thru and you see "try our new hot caramel cinnamon rolls." Who can resist that? You stroll down a grocery store aisle and see so many new cookie and dessert innovations that you could eat a different one every night. You turn on the TV and you are lured to try the latest crispy/melty/gooey/cheesy/chocolatey/chewy products. It goes on and on. The common thread is usually a bleached flour based carbohydrate or just a lot of sugar mixed with a large amount of fat (oil or butter). Fifteen years ago, most people had dinner and that was it. Now most people have dessert every night and a latte with a pastry at some point along the way.

The problem is that while your brain cells need carbs to function, your body can only handle a small amount of carbs at one time. So we need a strategy to make that fuel last longer and keep it from going into fat storage.

The best approach is not to starve yourself but to eat a reasonable amount at frequent intervals throughout the day. Not too much so that you overfeed your body's needs, but not too little so that you cause yourself to desire more later. The right amount of food (specifically, carbs) will elevate your blood sugar to an appropriate level, providing

Skinny Chick 10-Week Transformation

NAME: DIANNE M.
AGE: 31
TOTAL POUNDS LOST: 17.5
TOTAL INCHES LOST: 31.25

I've always had a mental projection of myself as a "big girl" ever since I was 9 years old and weighed about 100 pounds. Even when I was relatively small, my mental picture has always been of a big person who needed to cover herself up. The summer I was 9, my parents discovered the big warehouse clubs and started buying candy and chocolate bars in bulk. It made me feel really rich to be able to have this vast amount of food in my house. I really went out of control. When I started fourth grade, I was a lot plumper than I had been the year before—and I stayed that way. In high school and college I relied on baggy shirts and men's Levi's to hide my body.

For the past few years, I have basically had only one pair of pants that I felt comfortable wearing: size 11 cargo pants that covered everything. Since following the Skinny Chicks program, I have started to pull out things from my closet, and now I'm fitting comfortably into size 6 and size 8 pants; I've quadrupled my wardrobe options! I'm especially happy to have lost a lot of weight in my midsection because I had a real problem with that "muffin top" spilling out over my waistband.

I've tried other weight loss programs where I felt like I was really suffering and restricting calories, but Christine's program is special. I really like that Christine gave me a scientific program and explained how combining carbs and proteins and essential fats in our diets helps our bodies work better and more efficiently. She gave us the tools to be able to eat forever in a healthy way and not gain weight. I weighed and measured my food at the beginning of the program, but I soon learned the portion sizes for my meals. Now I know exactly what 4 ounces of chicken looks like, and exactly what a cup of brown rice looks like. For me, the key to this program is that you can do it with any food, in any place, at any supermarket, at any restaurant—not like other diets that make it difficult to go out into the world and live your real life.

I definitely feel healthier. I feel like my energy level has stabilized. When I started the program, I had come from a place where I was feeling guilty about everything I put in my mouth. Now I feel like I have the tools to know exactly how my body is processing food and exactly what it requires, so I don't need to give it more and I don't need to give it less. Christine has shown me that you don't need to starve to get the body you want.

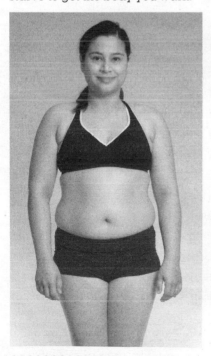 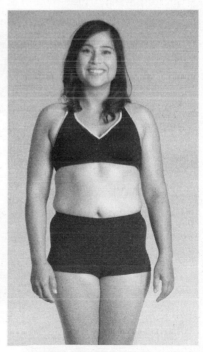

much-needed fuel for your brain and nervous system. If weight loss is the objective, you want to eat only enough to fuel the body's needs and no more, so there is no extra to be stored as fat. In this way, you actually feed your body all the nutrients it needs for energy, body function, immunity, skin, hair, and hunger satiation, so that your muscles can do the work of burning calories from fat all day and night.

So, What Is a Reasonable Amount?

What seems like a reasonable amount of food to me may be something entirely different to you. There has to be some objective standard. That standard exists in the form of calories. A calorie is, basically, a unit of energy. Human beings function—breathe, move, digest, pump blood—on energy. The number of calories any food contains tells us how much potential energy is in that food. When we eat, metabolic processes burn the fuel and turn it into molecular substances that can be put to immediate use by our cells, or stored away as fat.

So, from the nutritional point of view, a reasonable amount of food is the number of calories your cells need to function well. That number is different for every person.

How Do You Determine How Many Calories to Eat?

I recommend eating a consistent number of calories at breakfast, lunch, and dinner. As for snacks, you should be eating every 4 hours, so you may not need a midmorning snack, depending on your schedule. However, for most people, the gap between lunch and dinner stretches well beyond 4 hours; therefore, it is highly important to eat a midafternoon meal or snack, depending on your hunger level. Most women should be eating approximately 1,500 calories per day, and that is the approximate number of calories you'll find in each Skinny Chicks' meal plan.

If you don't know exactly how many calories a food contains, don't panic. I tell my clients to eat a protein such as a grilled salmon fillet or chicken breast about the size of their palm. Then I tell them to have a healthy carb such as rice pilaf or a sweet potato about the size of their clenched fist. A portion of fat should be approximately the size of a shot glass for nuts and $^1/_2$ a shot glass for oils. This is a rough estimate. A snack should be about half the size (and calories) of a regular meal.

The Source of Your Calories

In theory, one calorie is just like any other. Remember the old riddle—which is heavier, a pound of bricks or a pound of feathers? It's a trick question, because a pound is a pound is a pound. So, in theory, it shouldn't matter whether you eat carbs, protein, or fat, as long as the calories add up to the right number. It shouldn't matter whether you eat 500 calories of chicken or 500 calories of chicken fat. As long as someone eats 500 less calories per day, they should lose 1 pound per week according to "the numbers." (1 pound = 3,500 calories; 7 days × 500 calories = 3,500 calories.) But we're not purely talking numbers here; we're talking health as well. We're talking nutrition. So we want to set certain parameters for nutritional content that will keep our calories within a healthy, blood sugar–stabilizing range. To achieve this, we should consume a mix of carbohydrates, protein, and fat, in these proportions:

- 50 to 60 percent carbohydrates (approximately the size of 1$^1/_2$ fists)

- 25 to 30 percent proteins (approximately the size of your palm)

- 15 to 20 percent fats (approximately the size of a shot glass for nuts or $^1/_2$ shot glass for oils)

These are not percentages you want to add up at the end of the day; you want this balance at each and every meal. The body is not a cash register. The balance of nutrients you consume at every meal is the most crucial piece of the puzzle, and we will cover it in detail in the next chapter.

CHAPTER 4

The Beauty of Balance

Every trendy diet program has its "magic bullet." The Atkins diet had its "no carbs" rule, the Sugar Busters diet had no sugar, the cabbage soup diet had . . . well . . . cabbage soup. The Skinny Chicks program is not a diet; it is a healthy lifestyle nutrition program. Therefore it offers no magic bullet for weight loss. However, I do have a golden rule of eating, and it's as simple as it is effective: *Eat a combo of protein and carbs at every meal*. Why? Because it is the most effective way to stabilize blood sugar levels with food (aside from memorizing the glycemic index). Follow this straightforward guideline every time you eat, and I promise you that you will see results.

Dispelling the No-Carb Myth

There are three primary energy-yielding nutrients in our food: protein, carbs, and fats. These are known as macronutrients. Our bodies can break down these macronutrients into life-sustaining energy that can be used by our cells. But that's not all we need. We also need to consume vitamins and minerals (micronutrients) in order for the body to work; however, we do not obtain energy from micronutrients. Only protein, carbs, and fats give our bodies the energy we need to sustain life.

We now know that the carbs in our food are turned into glucose, which is in turn delivered by the insulin FatEx service. Some of that glucose is dumped into your bloodstream and used immediately by your cells for energy; some is converted into glycogen, the form of glucose that is stored in your muscles and liver; whatever is left over goes into storage and is, basically, what makes you fat (or fatter).

Unfortunately, many people reduce the entire study of nutrition down to two words: "No carbs." And these people are absolutely right. By cutting out carbs they *will* lose fat—along with their muscle tissue and their sanity.

What happens to a person who adopts the "no carb" mantra? You get the three-times-per-day cave-ins and the late-night sweet binges. You get overwhelming cravings for cookies you wake up in the middle of the night to eat. The body needs carbs and it doesn't care how it gets them. Sooner or later your body will win and get its carbohydrate fix— usually in an extra-large quantity.

Let's do another review of how our bodies respond to our real lives. Often, when we get on a health kick, we get up in the morning and have a nice, tall glass of ice-cold orange juice for breakfast. What could be healthier than a straight-from-the-Florida-sunshine breakfast? But when you drink the orange juice (a very sugar-rich carbohydrate) on an empty stomach, your blood sugar level rises rapidly and insulin rushes into the bloodstream. You feel energized because there is glucose in your system to feed your brain, but this rapid rise in blood sugar doesn't last. In a couple of hours you feel very hungry and fatigued. You go into a state known as brain fog, which can only be cured by a trained professional at Starbucks. If you miss your coffee break, look out! Around 11:00 a.m., your body rapidly releases adrenaline and you are in a state of near-panic hunger. You feel like a depraved madwoman as you grab a doughnut and cackle, "I've got you now, my pretty!" Most of us buy into the "I'm starving, so I must be losing weight" myth, but the truth is just the opposite. If all you've had was orange juice, coffee, and a doughnut, you have flooded your system with glucose, and it is possible that even this small breakfast caused some fat storage because you had too many carbs at once.

Suppose that instead of having only a glass of OJ for breakfast, you also have a delicious egg white scramble. With some protein in your system, your blood sugar level elevates more slowly. The presence of protein in a meal causes the body to prolong satiety and keep blood sugar stable longer than with a non-protein meal. You feel energized and alert—basically like a human being again. Furthermore, because you haven't had too much glucose flooding your bloodstream at once, you minimize the amount of excess being stored as fat and you feel satisfied instead of stressed out.

The PC Combo Solution

The simple solution is . . . eating a combination of protein and carbs with every meal. Skinny Chicks don't eat salads, they eat PC Combos!

It seems too simple to make a difference, but when you follow this rule consistently, you'll find that it makes a big difference. As with most successful couples, it's all about chemistry, and a protein/carb combo is a match made in heaven. Your blood sugar is stable when amino acids (proteins) accompany glucose (carbohydrates) while traveling through the bloodstream. The reason? Proteins naturally lower the glycemic index (rate of sugar release) of a carbohydrate. Thus, combining proteins with carbs helps stabilize blood sugar; prolongs energy and satiety; and makes weight loss so much easier.

If you're wondering where fats fit into all this, truth be told, fats also lower the glycemic index of a carbohydrate. But, here's my advice: The majority of us don't have to put a lot of thought and effort into making sure we consume the necessary amount of fat. We'll get our 20 percent with or without trying. Any effort you expend on the fat front should go into making sure you're getting enough "good" fats; more on that later. What's important to remember is that when it comes to meals or snack time, chow down on a PC Combo.

Merging Onto the Blood Sugar Freeway

Think about the insulin FatEx truck cruising through the bloodstream. I call it the Blood Sugar Freeway (BSF). Ever been in a hurry to get to the

Skinny Chick 10-Week Transformation

NAME: LEZLIE W.

AGE: 25

TOTAL POUNDS LOST: 1

TOTAL INCHES LOST: 1

EMOTION LOST: CHRONIC DEPRESSION

EMOTION GAINED: JOY AND HAPPINESS

(Sometimes it's not just about weight. Lezlie is a model and did not need to lose weight, but she was curious about nutrition, and her sessions with me changed the course of her life forever. Read on.)

I have suffered from anxiety and depression from early childhood. As I reached puberty, the hormones only made it worse. When I was at home, we usually ate spaghetti or some kind of chicken dish. When I was away from home, my diet consisted of sugar, sugar, and more sugar. I was always a skinny girl. All of the other girls were developing curves, and I was still a pole. At the time, I didn't appreciate it, and I remember doing things like eating pints of ice cream before bed in hopes of gaining a few extra pounds.

By the time I hit college, I finally gained a little weight and developed the curves I had dreamed about for years, only to find that the attention made me insecure rather than happy. I began a cycle of binge eating.

At the same time, I began to experience extreme mood fluctuations. I remember watching TV with a boyfriend one night: The sound from the bag of chips he was eating began to drive me crazy, so much so that I envisioned throwing him out of the window.

After college, I relocated to Los Angeles to pursue the arts full time. The first year in Hollywood was almost enough to send me packing home in tears. But somehow, by the grace of God, I made it through.

I turned to prescription drugs to help me gain some control over my depression and anxiety, which regularly caused me to miss auditions and classes. I went from a size 4, 125 pounds, to a size 8, and 142 pounds. During the months when I took medication, I felt extremely calm. However, those around me would mention that I wasn't "me." Apparently, I became a zombie. I didn't care, though; I'd rather be a zombie than a monster.

And then I began Christine's nutrition program. On the first day, when Christine listed the symptoms of hypoglycemia, I looked at her in wonder; could it be that I had been treating hypoglycemia with depression medication? No one had ever mentioned hypoglycemia to me before. And when I met with my psychologist, he never asked me about my eating habits, only about my emotional state.

I decided that if I began to feel better on Christine's program, I would transition off the medication. After 3 weeks of her regimen, I felt healthier than I ever had in my entire life. My mood was sunny; I had less "nerves." And, with the help of my doctor, I was able to wean myself off of my medicine. And I hope my story will encourage other women who suffer from depression and anxiety. After trying everything under the sun, it was this program that really helped me conquer my demons.

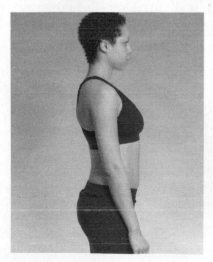 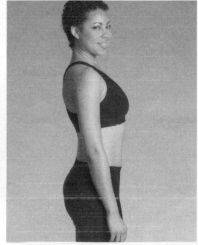

airport when the freeway is clogged with traffic? I have, and it isn't fun. But when you are on the freeway driving to the airport and there is no traffic, you zip right through in a matter of minutes. This is great if you're in a car. In your body, however, you actually *want* traffic on the Blood Sugar Freeway because when glucose (from carbs) is alone in the bloodstream, it zips right through to fat storage.

Let's go back to that morning glass of OJ for a moment. When you drink the juice, your body releases a fleet of insulin FatEx trucks to carry little packages of this new glucose to its trillions of cells. If your cells' glucose levels are low (which they are if you haven't eaten for more than 5 hours), the FatEx truck leaves a package of glucose in your cells. Once all the cells are full of energy/glucose, the FatEx truck dumps the extra glucose in the body's storage containers: fat cells. When the Blood Sugar Freeway is empty, the FatEx truck makes its deliveries so quickly that there is more glucose than your cells need, causing much to be stored as fat.

Now, let's imagine you had that egg white scramble with your orange juice. (Heck, while we're at it, let's scramble in some green onions, tomatoes, and cheese—a radical concept for us girls: a civilized breakfast.) Inside your body, the egg protein is broken down into amino acids that also enter the bloodstream. Now there's some traffic on the Blood Sugar Freeway, and it takes the FatEx truck longer to deliver its glucose packages. Protein is causing your body to release amino acids onto the Blood Sugar Freeway to help stabilize your blood sugar. This added traffic on the BSF helps your body receive glucose energy slowly over a period of hours, keeping your energy steady until lunchtime. When it comes to weight loss, your cells need a steady supply of glucose, not a glucose feast or famine. So even though traffic is the bane of your existence in real life, you actually want your insulin FatEx truck to be stuck in slow-moving traffic on the Blood Sugar Freeway.

The Balancing Act

Nutrition is not just about losing fat. It is also about getting all the vitamins and minerals (micronutrients) you need. The greater a variety of healthy foods you eat, the more likely it is that you will get enough vitamins and minerals. For that reason, you need to eat a balance of starchy, high-fiber carbs—whole wheat pasta, brown rice, whole grain bread—and nutrient-packed carbs—fruits and vegetables. Healthy starchy carbs give you more of the energy you need to survive, and they are packed with fiber (which helps to stabilize blood sugar), vitamins, minerals, and antioxidants.

Another reason to eat a balance of protein, carbs, and fats at every meal is that it is far more satisfying. When you eat this way, you feel like you're eating real, honest food because, well, you *are*. You have a nice feeling of fullness for a longer time. It's not the same lethargic, bloated feeling of fullness you get from eating 12 Krispy Kremes; it is a healthy, steady energy. Once my clients find out what is going on inside their bodies, they no longer feel so stressed out about their food choices. After 1 week on my program, a client told me she hadn't felt so relaxed about food and eating for 2 decades.

The Protein/Carb/Fat Formula

Now that you understand how important it is to have a PC Combo at every meal, you're probably wondering how much of the P to combine with the C. As a general rule, to maintain optimum blood sugar levels for weight loss, you should eat roughly two parts carbohydrates to one part protein. As we learned in the previous chapter, you should obtain 25 to 30 percent of your calories from lean protein sources. Roughly double this amount (50 to 60 percent) of your calories should come from healthy carbs, and the remainder (15 to 20 percent) should come from healthy fats. (For lists of lean proteins, healthy carbs, and good fats, see the Appendix starting on page 286.)

Remember that these are calorie measurements, not volume or weight measurements, so don't go and measure these out in a measuring cup or on a scale. Fats pack a very large number of calories in a very small space compared with carbohydrates or even most proteins. That's why a few pats of butter might have the same number of calories as an entire plate of pasta. The only way to get these calorie balances truly

DIVIDE YOUR PLATE

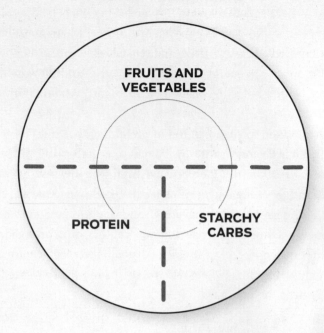

perfect is to read the labels of every food and add up the calories, and although this is tedious, I often counsel my clients to do just that, especially when beginning the program. The good news is that once you get the hang of it, you won't have to pay such meticulous attention to calorie counts and you can use your hand as a guide for portion control. For most people, the right balance looks like this: protein, such as grilled chicken breast, lean steak, or fish roughly the size of your palm; a delicious starchy, high-fiber carb such as pasta or rice, roughly the size of your closed fist; and two scoops of healthy vegetables. You can also think of it this way: Divide your plate into four and fill one quarter with protein. Fill another quarter with a starchy carb. The remaining two quarters should be filled with healthy fruits or vegetables (see the Appendix). Use a small amount (no more than a tablespoon) of healthy fats such as olive oil for cooking or additional flavor.

If you are still not sure how much you should be eating, check out the meal plans starting on page 122; they'll give you a lot of great meal ideas that don't require you to weigh or measure every item.

But beware of sticking to the letter of this healthy habit while ignoring the spirit behind it. For instance, I once had a client who loved jelly beans; she would literally eat a grilled chicken breast with a handful of these sweet little candies. Was she successful at dropping pounds? As a matter of fact, she was. But she was feeding her body a food that had absolutely no nutritional value whatsoever. Depriving your body of the nutrients it needs deprives you of living your best, healthiest life. Plus, if you don't nurture your body along the way, sooner or later you'll come up against a mountain of health problems. Eating a healthy balance means eating not only a PC Combo but also a variety of foods to get all the vitamins and minerals your body needs. If I were to help you succeed in losing weight but let you become sick due to vitamin deficiencies, I wouldn't be much of a nutritionist. So be adventurous and eat a wide variety of healthy foods.

CHAPTER 5

Munch around
the Clock

One, two, three o'clock, four o'clock munch.
Five, six, seven o'clock, eight o'clock crunch.
Nine, ten, eleven o'clock, twelve o'clock lunch.
We're gonna munch around the clock today!

In 1953, Bill Haley and the Comets had a revolutionary idea that went
against what most people thought of as "the norm." Haley wanted everyone to rock around the clock. Well, now it's time for another revolutionary rockin' idea: munch around the clock.

If you're eating to stabilize your blood sugar levels so that you can
lose weight and live your healthiest life, *when* you eat is just as important
as *what* you eat. When it comes to losing weight, most people try to eat
less often, and less food at each meal, thinking food deprivation is the
ticket to weight loss. They couldn't be more wrong! This chapter will
help ease that confusion.

Here's what you need to know: Skinny Chicks eat every 4 hours,
whether it's a complete meal or a snack. This will keep your blood sugar

at a consistent level. This doesn't mean have breakfast at 7:00 a.m. and lunch at 12:00 p.m.; it means if you eat your first meal at 7:00 a.m., have lunch at 11:00 a.m. Then have another lunch or a snack at 3:00 p.m. and eat dinner at 7:00 p.m. If you eat at 7:30 p.m. and you are up until 12:00 midnight, you should eat a PC Combo meal before bed. My clients do this all the time and still continue to lose weight. Of course if you are not that hungry, I recommend you eat a smaller meal . . . but you need to eat *something*. Of course I realize this is contrary to what people normally do in order to lose weight. However, on the Skinny Chicks program you *need* to eat every 4 hours in order to avoid those sugar binges.

If you eat only when you are ravenously hungry, you will have waited until your body is out of stored glucose. Your blood sugar level will be in the basement and you'll feel it. You'll lose your ability to concentrate, you'll feel lightheaded, and you'll likely experience physical hunger "pangs." And you know what happens then—you start to hear that voice in your head that says, "Eat! Eat!" And it's not saying, "Eat a big piece of fish." Your brain needs fuel and will work hard to convince you to go get the most carbohydrate-laden snack you can find.

Starving yourself sets you up to crave all the foods you *shouldn't* be eating. If, instead, you have a PC Combo every 4 hours, your blood sugar will love you for it and you'll set yourself up to choose the right foods.

The Clock Strikes "Carb"

Blood sugar levels drop dramatically 3 to 4 hours after a meal, regardless of the amount of carbohydrates previously consumed. If you had an overabundance of carbohydrates in your previous meal, just remember that the FatEx truck is busy riding around, delivering special packages in various places on your body, giving you more lumps, bumps, hips, and thighs than your body wants or needs.

It's when we are too busy to eat that we get into trouble. We get too involved in what we are doing, and we think we'll save time by hitting the vending machine. We tell ourselves, "I'm starving and I don't have time for a real meal, so I'll just have a handful of chips." What happens then? A handful turns into half the bag, and half the bag becomes the entire bag, and sometimes even that's not enough. Not long after, you notice that all the sodium from the chips has made you extremely thirsty, so you reach for a large soda. Why? First, when salt is absorbed into the bloodstream, it makes the fluid outside your cells saltier than the fluid inside your cells. That extra salt essentially calls out to the salt inside the cells and says, "Hey, come on out here and play." The cell, always the goody two-shoes and looking for balance, e-mails the brain and says, "There's too much salt floating around outside. Send me some help." That's when you start to feel thirsty. All that extra salt also increases the amount of electrolytes in our blood. Electrolytes carry the electrical impulses that help control our bodily functions. Too many electrolytes turns on the thirst center, and we need liquids to get us back in balance again. That's why, when you go into a bar, you'll often find peanuts, popcorn, or pretzels free for the taking. Those smart bar owners know that those salty snacks will have us ordering more drinks quicker than Shakira can shake her booty.

And that's also why we reach for something sweet to drink. We all know that sweet flavors taste phenomenal with salty flavors. So you grab a soda, and 750 calories later, you feel energized, yet puffy and borderline depressed.

It is far better to stop what you are doing for 5 minutes and prepare yourself a PC Combo, like a turkey sandwich or a bowl of fruit with cottage cheese. If you make this part of your daily routine, you won't get to the point where your body is craving the chips and sweets. You won't even miss them at all!

Why You Need to Eat Every 4 Hours

Imagine this scenario: You're a contestant on *Survivor: Skinny Chicks Island*. You haven't eaten anything but a few ugly bugs for 24 hours. Suddenly, you come across a wild bird sitting on a nest of six eggs. You quickly scoop them up and hide them in your pockets. You are tempted to eat all six at once, but your instincts tell you otherwise, so you eat one now and save the rest for later, one every few hours. That way you will spread out your energy resources as long as possible.

That's an extreme example, but you get the idea. If you ate all the eggs at once, you'd have consumed extra calories your body would not be able to use that would just go to waste (or to waist, as the case may be). This is essentially what happens when you eat three large meals a day with many hours in between each meal. By eating smaller meals every 4 hours, your body gets just the right amount of energy and uses it for the fuel it needs.

Many studies have shown that eating smaller, more frequent meals is not only better for losing weight, but better for your general health as well. One early study, published in 1989, divided participants into two separate groups. Both groups were given the same number of calories to consume each day, but one group ate a regular breakfast, lunch, and dinner while the second group was fed 17 small snacks throughout the day. At the end of the study, the "nibblers" had lowered their cholesterol by 14 percent and decreased their average insulin level by 28 percent.

Another study, from the *Proceedings of the National Academy of Sciences*, suggested that if you want to keep thinking, you've got to keep eating. Have you ever noticed that your ability to concentrate decreases as your hunger increases? You're not imagining things. The study found that " . . . cognitive ability can deplete extra-cellular glucose in the hippocampus . . . ," the region of the brain critical for learning and memory, and that " . . . exogenous glucose administration reverses the depletion while enhancing task performance." In other words, thinking is hard work that causes the brain to use up energy supplies faster than do other regions of the body during critical problem solving. The only way to get your cognitive abilities up to par once again is to feed the brain more glucose by having a snack or a meal. Obviously, the best way to keep your brain train on track at all times is to keep it continuously supplied with fuel *before it becomes depleted,* which means eating every 4 hours.

Here are some other reasons to munch around the clock:

- Muscle tissue is better preserved when you eat every 4 hours. This is good because more muscle means a faster metabolism.

- Liver tissue is preserved if you eat every 4 hours. This is good because a healthy liver also means a faster metabolism.

Skinny Chick Chat

Dear Christine: What happens when fat stores are used up? Where do those fat cells go?

JOANNE C., BATON ROUGE

Joanne: Actually, except for a small percentage of fat cells, they don't go anywhere. A new study reported in the *New York Times* found that every year, no matter how fat or thin you are, or whether you lose or gain weight, 10 percent of your fat cells die. However, every year the cells that die are replaced by new fat cells. The result is that the number of fat cells in your body remains the same throughout your adult life. Losing weight only affects the amount of fat stored in the cells, not the number of cells, and the same goes for gaining weight. Overweight people have more fat cells in their bodies than thin people do. Even people who have had weight loss surgery and lost hundreds of pounds possess the same number of fat cells they had before the surgery—even if they have become much thinner. One theory, called the fat cell hypothesis, says that the number of fat cells is determined early in life, and after that they can change only in size, not in number. When people lose weight and the fat cells shrink, the cells send hormonal signals asking to be filled up again. That's why most people regain weight that they have lost. Unfortunately, scientists are still searching for ways to turn off that signal. In the meantime, the best way to get those fat cells to shrink and "stay shrunk" is to follow the Skinny Chicks program.

EAT WELL, CHRISTINE

- The brain needs a constant, steady stream of glucose for survival. Brain cells use up to twice as much blood sugar as any other cell in the body.

- It's nice to eat often. Who doesn't like to eat?

Running on Empty

When a car runs out of gas and conks out, it just stops moving. There is no reserve tank it can switch to for more fuel. Remember that when we humans run out of fuel (blood sugar—Tank 1), we don't conk out because we do have reserve tanks: glycogen in liver and muscle tissue (Tank 2), our lean tissues and organs (Tank 3), and body fat (ketosis—Tank 4). The body doesn't conk out like a car because it starts eating through its own engine. If you are running on nothing but caffeine all day, you are borrowing energy from your own body. But that's good, isn't it? Don't we want to burn our own body fat for energy?

Unfortunately, the body doesn't work that simply. This is why there are so many overweight people and also why so much money is poured into the industry of weight-loss advice. After glucose from food runs out, your body accesses some body fat, but it goes after glycogen stored in your liver tissue first. Then, after a few more hours, your body begins to convert muscle tissue to glucose (a process called glycogenolysis, the biochemical breakdown of glycogen to glucose). Now your metabolism slows to a crawl and fat burning in your body is minimized. Furthermore, you are starving and you feel like a miserable crankmizer. Only after about 24 to 72 hours (depending on the individual) does your body begin to significantly access body fat for energy. But as we observed in Chapter 3, there are very few of us who can actually hold out for a full 3 days without eating (or simply without eating carbs). If you are strong-willed enough to get through the 72 hours of carb deprivation, you will lose weight. But before you go on a hunger strike, remember this: Your metabolic rate will also be slower because your muscle and liver tissues will have been compromised. Worst of all, you will gain back most if not all of the weight once you begin to eat "real" food again.

Skinny Chick 10-Week Transformation

NAME: RAHA T.

AGE: 20

TOTAL POUNDS LOST: 16

TOTAL INCHES LOST: 22.5

When I was young, I was really, really thin—so thin that my ribs stuck out. Then puberty came along and so did a tire around my waist. I was the only kid around with big boobs and a big stomach. I always felt like the biggest girl in the room.

I was a compulsive dieter, but nothing really worked. I suffered from depression and anxiety, and that made me lose weight, but 5 minutes later I would gain it back again. I was stuck in a compulsive dieting/eating cycle.

What I learned from Christine's program is that starvation doesn't work, and it's okay to have carbs. You need carbs to sustain your life. And I learned that you need to combine protein and carbs, so I can have chicken and rice for dinner, which I love, and it's been working.

This program has actually created a lot of balance in my life because of the scheduling. I'm now eating really good food every 4 hours. When the 4 hours are up, I can't wait to eat my yogurt and fruit, or whatever I'm having. My life is now scheduled around these 4-hour intervals, and it works perfectly. When I went shopping and bought my first batch of food, it all fell into place for me, and it was easy breezy from there!

By week 3, I was already looking different and people were asking if I had lost weight. I slept really well at night and found I woke up even before my alarm went off. I don't have cravings anymore. And not only that—people have seen a significant difference in my attitude. I'm not as moody. I've never been so happy.

Several days without adequate food would mean a tremendous metabolic slowdown. The fat inside each fat cell cannot get out and actually leave your body in a healthy and permanent way unless you can keep the Blood Sugar Freeway moving. It wants out but everything has come to a screeching halt, because if you do not eat frequent meals, your body will hold on to stored fat and slow down cellular processes in an effort to conserve fuel/energy.

Midnight Munchies

Now, I'm not going to ask you to get up in the middle of the night to continue the every-4-hours pattern. You don't need as much energy while you're sleeping, and your body will dip into its reserve fuel sources to get what it does need. But you must eat breakfast within 1 hour of waking. And if you eat every 4 hours during the day, your blood sugar will be stabilized throughout the day and your hormones will be more balanced, which aids sleep. Furthermore, sleeping for 8 hours actually helps your body keep weight off, so you should spend your nights in dreamland instead of foodland. The good news is that you won't be hungry at night because you have eaten solid, fulfilling PC Combo meals throughout the day and into the evening.

CHAPTER 6

Every Body's Got Issues

Okay. Here's another pop quiz, and this one's a doozy.

- Quick—without thinking about it, name five parts of your body you truly love.
- Now, without thinking about it, name five parts of your body you can't stand.

Which one of those lists was easier to make? I can almost guarantee it was the second one, and I wouldn't be surprised if you came up with more than five. It's a sad fact of the world we live in today that we judge ourselves and our imperfections so harshly. Even the skinniest of chicks has areas that make her unhappy. We are embarrassed to be in our own skins.

Through my experience with thousands of clients, I've learned that people cannot lose weight successfully if they are in the midst of an internal battle. One of two things will happen:

1. They will lose the weight out of self-hate and disgust, which often becomes an eating disorder, or

2. When they do make progress and lose weight, they will allow negative thoughts to steal their joy and tell them that they really have not progressed, which brings self-defeat and sends them into a binge eating frenzy.

You Are What You Think

Many health gurus say "you are what you eat," which is somewhat true; however, my mantra is "you are what you think." A large portion of my nutrition consulting appointments are spent explaining to my clients that they must change their thoughts about themselves before they can succeed with weight loss. If they think of themselves as fit and healthy, it will become reality.

I can tell you that on this program you will lose weight and have more energy within the first week. I can also tell you that if you continue to let negative thoughts about your body into your mind, you will have a very difficult time losing weight. I've seen these thoughts drive away my clients' hopes of ever improving their shape and health. It's as if the body senses your view of yourself and makes it reality by not allowing the weight to come off. After years of dealing with both people who are overweight and those who are in wonderful shape, I've learned that our thoughts and words hold the power to keep us where we are or get us where we want to go. So, before you begin my weight loss program, I would like you to make an effort to release all the negative thoughts you have about your body and begin to use healthy thoughts and healthy words in your life. You need healthy thoughts to inspire healthy actions.

I know all about body issues. I was a runway model at 12, a bathing suit model in my teens, and in my early twenties, I appeared on the cover of fitness magazines. To be a successful fitness model, you have to be lean, cut, chiseled—flawless. You can't go to a photo shoot with your stomach protruding even a tiny bit, so you don't eat breakfast. You don't eat lunch. By 3:00 in the afternoon, you're ready to faint—but you don't dare eat. You're standing there as a representation of perfect health while you're actually dying inside because your body is breaking down muscle

Skinny Chick Chat

Dear Christine: I've been following the Skinny Chicks program for several weeks now and making progress. But my friend Sheila, who's also on the program, is losing weight faster than I am. Last week, she lost 4 pounds and I only lost a pound and a half. What am I doing wrong?

JANINE F., SALT LAKE CITY

Here's my advice to you, Janine: Stay in your own lane. Don't look at the person next to you to see how well you're doing. A pound and a half in a week is fantastic! In the first few weeks of the Skinny Chicks test group, several of the women were constantly comparing themselves with others in the group. One woman, who had lost 2 pounds that week, went to the back of the room and cried when she saw that another woman had lost 5 pounds. I explained to her that everyone is different and that she shouldn't be disappointed in herself or think that she hadn't done the program correctly. Even if you don't lose any weight in a particular week, the simple fact that you're no longer going to a fast-food restaurant for lunch or having a bag of chips for dinner is something to celebrate. Keep track of your own progress, and allow yourself to feel good about it. You worked hard for those 2 pounds! Enjoy your accomplishment.

EAT WELL, CHRISTINE

and liver tissue in order to survive. You do whatever you need to do to keep that perfect body perfect. And all the while, you think you're fat.

When I was 5 feet 9 inches and 118 pounds, I struggled with negative body image. I thought I was defective and deformed. Imagine how I felt when I was 155 pounds, and everything in between. I knew I was unhealthy and I never felt good about myself. But the moment I learned the ABCs of nutrition, all of my negative body image thoughts went away. Once I understood how to eat for health, I somehow found peace and calm. Knowing how food and our hormones work internally gave me self-assurance that I was on my way. And it was at that moment that the body image issues went away forever. It was truly a miracle from God. I weighed 155 pounds, and for the first time in my life, I loved myself and my body just as it was. I knew I had a way to go to reach my desired weight, but I found peace in knowing how to get there healthfully. I didn't care how long it took; I was just happy to be at peace in my own skin. I hope and pray that this book will offer the same peace to you.

Balance, Blood Sugar, and Body Image

How was I able to turn my attitude around? By calling a truce between my mind and my body. When I was eating just ice cream, or subsisting on salads during the day and binge foods at night, my blood sugar was so out of whack that it was literally making me crazy. Once I began to understand the concept of the PC Combo and eat healthy foods, I could think clearly. The moodiness and depression began to recede, allowing me to develop a more realistic and accepting perspective on my own body.

Being out of balance causes the vicious cycle that makes you overeat and then hate yourself and then eat more and then hate yourself even more and then starve yourself and start all over again. When you learn to stabilize your blood sugar, you eliminate the cravings and the craziness that precipitate all the negative self-talk. You can learn to love the body you have, and, if you so choose, find the "skinny" that's best for you in a smart, healthy way. If you love your life and love your body, you will want to take care of it. We all know how much effort it takes to eat a healthy meal or to get yourself to the gym when everything seems hopeless. However, if you follow the Skinny Chicks program, balanced meals and moderate exercise will become a fundamental part of your overall lifestyle philosophy, and you will begin almost immediately to feel better about yourself. Instead of seeing yourself in a negative light, you will develop a fundamental identification with health and a love of life, just as I have.

Skinny Chick 10-Week Transformation

NAME: MELIDA N.

AGE: 20

TOTAL POUNDS LOST: 11

TOTAL INCHES LOST: 20.5

Growing up, I was never really fat—I've always been the "chubby" one. But I never felt like I fit in, especially because I was brought up in Germany, where everyone was tall, skinny, and blonde. I was constantly teased at school.

My mother was very conscious of my weight. She had always been thin, and she made a point of telling me that I was not. She started putting me on diets when I was 9, and she signed me up for every sport she could find. When you are 9 and your mom is telling you in an indirect way that you're not good enough, it affects your body image. You feel that your mother is disappointed or is ashamed of you. By the time I was 12, I had an eating disorder. It began when my mom put me on a diet that had you drink vinegar before every meal. I would take some before breakfast, and by the time I got to school, I had to throw up. My mother thought the diet was really working. She was happy because I was losing weight, not realizing what I was doing. Then I found out that a cousin was doing the same thing, so I thought, "It must be okay because other people are doing it too."

I came to the United States in 2000, where I literally got introduced to a different world. Here, people are more accepting of who you are—different shapes and sizes and different cultures. And my cousins here weren't all super skinny. I started to realize that even if I was gaining my mom's acceptance, it really wasn't good for me. I was tired all the time. I was getting sick more often.

Christine's program helped me get over my eating disorder and bad eating habits by showing me that I can eat every 4 hours and have great food that I love, and still lose weight and be healthy. She showed me that I don't have to hate food. Food is not my enemy. I can love food and be healthy.

Christine stresses to listen to your body. A lot of times I haven't been. I wasn't good to my body when it was telling me not to starve myself. I think that phrase is really important: *Love your body, listen to your body.* It's inspiring because you see results. When people give you compliments, it boosts your self-esteem. That's really important in how you carry yourself and how you look at life. Because of this program, I'm thinking things like *I can go to med school, I can lose weight, I can live a better life.* It's really exciting.

Stop Comparing and Start Dreaming Big

Body image issues are exacerbated when we compare ourselves with others, whether it's friends and family, actresses or models. There is no one who compares to you. There will always be people who are thinner, or richer, or more successful than you—at this time. Tomorrow, you may be at the top of the heap. Either way, what matters is that you believe in yourself and your self-worth no matter what anyone else has, does, or achieves.

Adopt a mind-set that says "I'm a Skinny Chick" even if you're not. If you have a mind-set that says "I'm always going to be overweight and unattractive and I'm never going to be anything different than that," guess what? That's what you're going to get. If it's not in your heart, it's not really going to make a difference in your life. You have to believe it.

PART II

SKINNY CHICKS

REVISIT PROTEIN

AND CARBS

CHAPTER 7

Lean, Mean Protein

Growing up, I remember Sunday afternoon dinners on my grandparents' ranch in Gilroy, California. By noon, the house was filled with smells of a traditional Italian family dinner: fresh, homemade Italian pasta with a savory red meat sauce. My grandmother used meats of every sort in her sauce: chicken, turkey, beef, pork, or even fish and seafood. The smell of the meat—sautéing in the onions, garlic, and spices— wafted throughout the house and drifted outside, where I was playing with my cousins. Before long, my large extended family would be lining up at the table. The meal was delicious and incredibly satisfying to all of us kids after playing outside all day.

It never occurred to me to wonder whether it was a healthy meal, or how I could eat and eat my grandmother's pasta and never gain a pound, even as I got older.

Eventually, I moved to San José in pursuit of the excitement of the big city and forgot all about the simplicity of youth. Somewhere in the 1980s and 1990s, pasta became a forbidden treat and Italian food was seen as old-fashioned and passé. Pizza, pasta Alfredo, even good old spaghetti were considered health *faux pas*. For a short while in the mid 1990s, the accepted wisdom in health and nutrition circles was to cut out pasta entirely.

Maybe that's why—get ready for a big revelation—I cook a huge pasta dinner for myself and my husband and any guests we might have every Sunday night. While I'm sautéing the meat, the incredible, savory aromas of onions, garlic, hot peppers, and extra virgin olive oil fill the whole house. I always add chicken, shrimp, salmon, or extra lean ground turkey meat, or sometimes turkey sausage as a treat for my husband. Whichever I choose, the primary element is the protein, and the most important part of the preparation is browning the meat. If you just add spice to meat after it is cooked, it will wash off in the sauce and end up tasting bland. However, if you sauté your meat with spices, the meat will burst with flavor in your mouth and it will make all the difference.

So, on Sunday nights we eat pasta to our heart's content, and yes, Mick Jagger, you *can* get satisfaction, because this dinner is fulfilling and satisfying. And it's not because of the pasta or the tomatoes; it's because of the protein. And that's the subject of this chapter: protein.

Almost everything we think of when we think of our bodies is made from protein: our cells, tissues, and organs; our hair, skin, blood, bones, and muscles. Protein is one of the three nutrients (along with fats and carbs) that provide calories to the body—4 calories per gram, in fact. At the end of this chapter, you'll find a list of the healthiest sources of protein for the Skinny Chicks program.

Here's what protein does for your metabolism:

- It helps stabilize blood sugar, enabling you to burn more fat between meals.

- It keeps you feeling fuller longer and minimizes the munchies.

- It slows the absorption and digestion of sugars (carbohydrates) and can lower the glycemic index of high glycemic index carbs (more on the glycemic index in Chapter 8).

- It helps maintain muscle mass, which keeps metabolism humming.

The Real Skinny
on Protein and Belly Fat

Researchers at the Royal Veterinary and Agricultural University in Copenhagen found that women and men who consumed at least 25 percent of their daily calories as protein lost 10 percent more belly fat than those who consumed just 12 percent of their calories as protein. This is important news, because belly fat is a danger sign of poor health. It turns out this kind of fat (called visceral fat) releases harmful hormones, turns into cholesterol in the bloodstream (which eventually turns into artery-clogging plaque), secretes substances that cause inflammation, and decreases the body's sensitivity to insulin. Although researchers are not exactly sure why eating more protein reduces belly fat, one theory says that it's possible that protein intake may trigger smaller releases of the stress hormone cortisol, which directs the body to store fat in the tummy area. Less cortisol, less muffin top!

By now, you know that the mainstay of the Skinny Chicks program is the PC Combo. But do you know why we need to include protein in every meal and snack? Because in order to deliver the benefits above, your body needs a constant supply. And while we can store fats and carbs for future use, we can't store protein. There's no reserve storage facility in the body to replenish the supply, so we have to keep a steady stream coming.

That doesn't mean you should be eating huge amounts of protein every day. We know that adults need a minimum of 0.8 gram of protein per day for every kilogram of body weight (1 kilogram = 2.2 pounds) just to keep from slowly breaking down their own tissues, although I recommend a little more than this. Remember that a serving size of protein is about the size of your palm. In fact, a few ounces of protein go a long way, so there's no need to overdo.

More Benefits of Protein

For a woman, protein is the thing that you want the most for the things most important to you: your skin and your hair. There is not a woman (or a man, for that matter) who doesn't want healthy skin and hair. Your skin and hair (along with your muscles, the hemoglobin in your blood, and many enzymes that keep you alive) are made up mostly of protein. Your body takes the proteins you eat, breaks them down into amino acids (the building blocks of proteins), recombines them into new proteins, and makes new skin cells and promotes hair growth. They also create antibodies that fight off infection and disease. If you deprive yourself of protein for a long time, you can say good-bye to healthy skin and hair because there will be no new building blocks for generating new hair and skin cells.

PROTEIN AND WEIGHT LOSS

From a weight-loss standpoint, there are many benefits to protein:

- The most important benefit is that protein creates a hormonal response that triggers fat burning.

- Protein eaten together with carbohydrates will slow the absorption of glucose (sugar from carbs) into the bloodstream, which will keep blood sugar levels more stable and provide steady healthy energy.

- A meal is always much more satisfying when it includes a lean portion of chicken, turkey, fish, or beef. And there are plenty of great vegetarian protein sources, too, such as low-fat soy foods like tofu and tempeh, low-fat yogurts and cheeses, and legumes—especially lentils (for a more complete list of vegetarian proteins, see page 286). When you feel sated, you are less inclined to snack between meals.

- When prepared correctly, meats are delicious, which is perhaps the most important thing of all, since you should love what you eat.

How does protein affect fat burning? Protein-rich meals trigger the release of the hormone glucagon, the antagonist hormone of insulin. As you know by now, insulin is a "storing" (anabolic) hormone. On the other hand, glucagon is a "mobilizing" (catabolic) hormone. Insulin clears away glucose and packs it away into cells for storage. Glucagon's job is to release glucose from cells when blood sugar levels are too low. According to Balint Kacsoh, MD, PhD, author of *Endocrine Physiology*, glucagon also stimulates lipolysis (the breakdown of fat for energy) in adipose tissue (fat) by activating hormone-sensitive lipase. In other words, glucagon is part of a process that ultimately helps break down triglycerides, which are stored body fats, into their component parts: free fatty acids and glycerol. Once these parts are separated, they can leave the fat cell and be used by the body for energy. This effect is subtle yet important, so please do not use this as a green light to load up on protein—remember, healthy weight loss is about eating PC Combos and not protein alone.

Which Proteins to Choose

The short answer is chicken, turkey, fish, egg whites, and low-fat/nonfat dairy products. I eat one of these in nearly every meal, and there are innumerable delicious ways to prepare each of them. (See the recipes starting on page 237.) If you are vegetarian or vegan, there are plenty of great choices for you as well (see page 286). If you want to lose weight, you want the leanest proteins, which are those listed above. Then you want to prepare them in a way that doesn't turn them into an oil sponge.

I recommend eating beef no more than once a week due to its high saturated fat content. The leanest cuts are those that include the word "loin," such as tenderloin or sirloin. If you enjoy steak, I say go ahead and throw a nice sirloin on the grill once a week. Pork is another lean meat for which it's best to choose the "loin" cuts for pork that is organically raised. Here are some other popular protein choices:

- **Chicken and turkey:** Most of my clients eat a large amount of chicken and turkey. Think beyond the Thanksgiving dinner. You can buy great-tasting turkey burgers, and you can replace ground beef with ground turkey in most recipes—often, the result is even tastier than the original. Enchiladas, burgers, pasta with meat sauce or meatballs, meat loaf, tacos, and even lasagna can all be made with turkey. Chicken can be sautéed in garlic, onions, and spices to provide the flavor base for dozens of great pasta and rice dishes that will not only fill you up but also taste so good they'll knock your socks off. And of course, if you are not inclined toward the kitchen, you can always throw chicken on the grill or buy a rotisserie chicken.

- **Fish:** Fish is a very lean source of protein. I don't think there is any food in the world that I love more than Chilean sea bass, but due to its high price and endangered status, it's an infrequent treat for me and most folks. Close favorites include salmon, halibut, orange roughy, scallops, and shrimp. Sushi with salmon, eel, crab, and shrimp are healthy choices as well as delicious. Tuna is a great protein source, though I recommend moderation due to the possibility (albeit small) of trace mercury content. I tell my clients to limit tuna to one 3-ounce serving per week. (The FDA says that it is safe for pregnant women to consume two 6-ounce servings of light tuna per week, but I often advise women who are pregnant or planning on becoming pregnant to avoid all tuna until after they finish breastfeeding.)

- **Eggs:** Eggs are a great source of protein, and there is nothing more satisfying and long-lasting than a hot breakfast with eggs. I always use egg whites with just a little yolk, as the yolks are high in cholesterol and fat. One egg yolk has approximately 4 grams of fat, so it's not the best choice for people who want to lose weight, but egg whites are a great lean source of protein, yielding 3 grams per white.

- **Dairy products:** Dairy products can be deceptive because they offer proteins, carbs, and fats in one bite, and they can vary in their protein content. It can present a bit of a challenge for meal preparation. The chart shows that not all yogurt is created equal:

TYPE OF YOGURT	CALORIES PER 6-OZ SERVING	PROTEIN (G)	CARBS (G)	FAT (G)	GOOD/BAD PROTEIN SOURCE?
Plain low-fat	75	11	16	2	Good source of protein
Greek, plain low-fat	110	15	7	3	Good source of protein
Plain, whole milk	130	8	11	6	Bad protein source—too much fat
Flavored, low-fat	157	7	30	1.5	Bad protein source—too many carbs
Flavored, whole milk	172	8	23	5	Bad protein source—you need 3 servings to get enough protein, thus too many carbs and too much fat
Greek, flavored, whole milk	283	9	32	14	Bad protein source—too much fat and carbs
Greek, plain, whole milk	221	12	5	17	Bad protein source—too much fat

*Comments based on recommended nutrition parameter of 1 part protein, 2 parts carbohydrates.

Magazine Article Diets

In virtually any magazine on the newsstand, you will find an article offering a quick slim-down diet from doctors known and unknown, fitness trainers, nutritionists, health experts, writers, and every other possible person under the sun with a computer. They inevitably recommend the following diet: Cereal with milk for breakfast, bagel with peanut butter for a snack, chicken salad for lunch, a handful of nuts for a snack, and a dinner of fish and vegetables. They add up the total protein, carbs, and fats for the day and presto: They suggest this is a balanced diet. But

Skinny Chick Chat

Dear Christine: I heard that I should stay away from fish because of the possibility of mercury. Can you tell me which types of fish are safe?

TAMIKA, DALLAS

Tamika: Your concerns about mercury are valid, but don't throw the baby out with the bathwater. The benefits of fish far outweigh the risks for most individuals. For children and for women who are of childbearing age, or who are pregnant or nursing, mercury is definitely a concern. Mercury, which comes from industrial emissions, burning coal, and natural sources, can harm a developing brain and nervous system. Fish that are high in mercury include shark, swordfish, king mackerel, and tilefish (also called golden snapper or golden bass). Another fish to avoid if you are of childbearing age is albacore tuna, which contains more mercury than light tuna does. (Canned tuna is the most widely consumed fish in our country.) I recommend swapping albacore tuna for light tuna and limiting yourself to one serving per week. It is, however, important for everyone to consume at least three 4-ounce servings of fish per week, according to the FDA, so you should still enjoy a variety of wild-caught fresh fish and shellfish. Some of the best are catfish, Pacific cod, Pacific halibut, pollock, salmon, tilapia, and trout. (Getting enough omega-3 fatty acids—of which fish are an excellent source—also aids a baby's nervous system development. Be sure to ask your doctor or OB-GYN for the latest recommendations on fish consumption.)

For more information on mercury in our fish, go to www.cfsan.fda.gov/~dms/admehg3.html.

EAT WELL, CHRISTINE

The Real Skinny
on Dairy's Weight-Loss Secrets

According to two research studies from the University of Tennessee's Nutrition Institute, calcium in dairy products can offer a mega-boost to your weight loss strategy. In one study, 32 obese women and men who cut 500 calories from their usual daily intake lost more weight when they added 800 milligrams of supplemental calcium daily. They also shed more fat when they were put on a diet that included 1,200 to 1,300 milligrams of calcium. In the other study, 34 obese people on a diet that included three servings of yogurt a day lost more body fat than a similar group who had only one serving.

your body doesn't add things up at the end of the day. It digests the food that's in your stomach at any given moment. I cringe whenever I see all these lightweight meals and snacks. For instance, a bowl of cereal with milk contains a small amount of protein (in the milk), but it's mostly refined carbs. It is neither satisfying nor a truly balanced meal, as there simply is not enough protein. The same goes for a bagel and peanut butter—you are getting a bunch of refined carbs and twice as much fat as protein.

A meal like that might stabilize blood sugar because there is fat and protein in peanut butter, but it won't satisfy your hunger. You feel like you are starving, because you are. Invariably you end up eating a huge dinner to compensate for the daylong deprivation—a dinner with second helpings, two glasses of wine, and a few desserts. Remember that weight gain happens when you take in too much at once and overwhelm the body with too many calories. The whole day of deprivation might cause a small amount of fat burning, but the big dinner will more than make up for it in fat storage. You may not have a massive binge the first night, but give it a few days and it is sure to happen.

The Real Skinny on Bagels for Breakfast

A study from the Rochester Center for Obesity Research in Michigan monitored 30 women who started their day with eggs and toast. The women felt so full and satisfied that they ate 274 fewer calories the rest of the day than those who had bagels and cream cheese for breakfast.

The best thing to do is spread the calories from the big dinner into the other three meals of the day. Remember the ABCs—especially your "Cs," because eating every 4 hours is extremely important if you seriously want to lose weight and keep it off. Make every meal you have a balanced meal that includes a healthy protein.

What If You Don't Eat Meat?

Plenty of people do not eat any animal proteins for reasons of personal preference or ethics. Your body doesn't take politics into account, though—it just reacts to the nutrients it receives. Proteins are a tremendously important part of everyone's diet, including vegetarians'. Fortunately, plant-based proteins such as tempeh, seitan, tofu, edamame, lentils, split peas, and kidney beans can provide many of the benefits you need without ever harming an animal. In addition, some vegetarians are open to eating fish, which, as I mentioned earlier, is a great protein source.

My message to vegetarians is the same one I give all my clients: Combine a protein with a carb at every meal. You might be thinking to yourself, "Well, beans are a carbohydrate *and* a protein, so is it okay for me to consider foods such as lentils a prefab carbohydrate-protein combo?" My answer is yes; however, vegetable protein sources are often higher in calories and even fat, so invest some time in learning their nutritional values.

Vegans, unlike vegetarians, eat no meat, eggs, or dairy. However, it is really difficult to satisfy your body's nutritional needs from veggie proteins alone, because many of the sources of plant proteins such as soybeans, nuts, and legumes are nutritionally lacking in one way or another. There are many benefits to eating soy, but recent research compiled by the Harvard School of Public Health finds that the benefits might be counterbalanced by the potential risks of consuming too *much*. One study uncovered a possible link to increased risk for certain cancers. Harvard recommends soy in moderation with an upper limit of four servings per week.

Of all the plant-based proteins, legumes are the best because they are a complete protein and there are no known adverse effects from eating them every day. Legumes include beans (e.g., garbanzo, lima, fava, navy, kidney, pinto, and black), peas (e.g., split, yellow, and green), and lentils. In places like India, where many people are vegetarians, legumes are a staple food.

In my practice in Los Angeles, I've worked with many vegans. One basically vegan client by the name of Nichole signed up for my "Fit and Lean Vegetarian" program and had tremendous success. Here is Nichole's story. This information has been taken directly out of Nichole's original files and has not been altered:

Nichole H., Manhattan Beach, California

Starting: 155 lbs, 22% body fat, size 12, 34 lbs fat, 120.9 lbs muscle

Ending: 143 lbs, 15% body fat, size 5, 22.4 lbs fat, 120.6 lbs muscle

The impressive thing to notice here is that she lost 12 pounds of body fat and zero pounds of muscle on this program and she dropped seven sizes! That should tell you that the numbers on a scale are not always the best indicator of a fit and lean person. On page 76 is an example of Nichole's vegetarian diet before she began working with me.

Food Log for Wednesday, March 29, 2006

(This is before she started the program.)

TIME OF MEAL	NICHOLE'S FOOD/ FEELING	CALORIES	CHRISTINE'S COMMENTS
7:30 a.m.	Breakfast bar . . . *still hungry*	150	Not enough protein or calories; this spikes blood sugar.
8:00 a.m.	Soy vanilla latte . . . *feeling okay*	160	Another high-sugar, low protein food; this spikes blood sugar.
10:00 a.m.	Apple . . . *starving*	120	Again, more carbs, some fiber, no protein; this will keep you hungry.
12:40 p.m.	4 gummy gators . . . *starving but hoping that sugar will pick me up*	35	Another blood sugar spike; this will keep you hungry.
1:15 p.m.	Sandwich made with wheat vegan bread, veggie meat (2 slices), and provolone cheese; lettuce, tomato, and honey mustard dressing; fake chicken meat pasta salad	680	This looks okay, but fake chicken salad probably has too much fat.
2:00 p.m.	Two pieces of hard candy	45	Blood sugar spike
3:00 p.m.	Handful of almonds and 4 pieces of chocolate	180	If you had had a complete breakfast this morning, you would not be reaching for candy; nuts are very high in fat. You should be eating a balanced meal here if you do not plan on having dinner until 8 p.m.
4:00 p.m.	Diet Coke; *I have one every afternoon*	Zero	Soda contains phosphates that have been shown to deplete bone mass.
6:30 p.m.	Quiznos veggie sandwich	230	If you had cheese and mayo, chances are that there is too much fat in the meal; this is also too low in protein . . . not enough food.
9:45 p.m.	Extra-large chocolate chip cookie	210	A cookie is okay once in a while if it's eaten after a balanced meal, but alone it will not satisfy the body's needs.

Here is a one-day sample menu that I created for Nichole after she started the program:

TIME OF MEAL	NICHOLE'S FOOD/ FEELING	CALORIES	CHRISTINE'S COMMENTS
Breakfast 7:00 a.m.	4 egg whites, 1 oz fat-free soy cheese, 1 cup pineapple, 1 slice Ezekiel bread spread with 100% natural fruit spread. *Feeling kinda full yet energized.*	310	Eaten within 1 hour of waking up. This meal is a good balance of proteins and high-fiber carbs, thus it will hold her over for approximately 4 hours.
Lunch 11:00 a.m.	Veggie cheese sandwich: 3 slices fat-free veggie cheese, cucumbers, sprouts, shredded carrot, spinach, tomato, spread with avocado and fat-free cream cheese and a medium pear. *Lots of energy, and I'm in a good mood.*	410	Eaten 4 hours later, this is another fantastic healthy PC Combo. She will be satisfied until at least 3:00.
Lunch #2 3:00 p.m.	Edamame and lentil salad with brown rice and artichoke hearts (canned in water), fat-free Italian dressing. *This was delicious and I'm surprised that I'm not craving sugar.*	410	Eaten 4 hours after the last meal. She is sure to be burning fat and saving muscle because her blood sugar is stable.
Dinner 7:00 p.m.	Low-fat tofu stir-fry—mixed veggies cooked with cooking spray, soy sauce, and citrus juice—and a side of brown rice. *This was good and I'm full; I can't even think of eating anything for the rest of the evening.*	330	Eaten 4 hours later. She will continue to have stable blood sugar levels and feel great throughout the evening.

"Before" meal totals: 1,810 calories, 82 grams protein, 271 grams carbs, 54 grams fat

"After" meal totals: 1,460 calories, 83 grams protein, 240 grams carbs, 21 grams fat

Nichole had been trying to lose 10 pounds for 2 years with no success before she came to me. Her goal was to eat less and exercise more to lose weight, but her weight loss strategy never worked because she was constantly hungry. As you see from her "before" food log, her meals were not PC Combos, and thus, her blood sugar would constantly spike. She'd stay hungry all day without ever feeling satisfied.

Nichole suffered from lack of energy, caffeine cravings, and mood swings, and her weight would not budge no matter what exercise or diet she tried. After we applied the ABCs to her eating habits, the stubborn pounds of fat began to melt away. In the beginning, Nikki was not happy about spending the extra time to cook and plan her food for each day, but after a few weeks she got the hang of it. She would come into my office perky and excited to share with me all of the new veggie proteins she had discovered. She created a shopping list of her favorite quick veggie protein/carb foods, and after she got into the routine of grocery shopping and preparing her meals, it became a piece of cake. In the end, Nikki lost 12 pounds of body fat and maintained all of her muscle without eating one piece of meat. I believe she is an inspiration to vegetarians everywhere.

Short Protein List (for a more detailed protein list, see the Appendix)

EAT AS OFTEN AS YOU LIKE

- Chicken
- Turkey
- Fish (not including tuna, shark, swordfish, king mackerel, and tilefish)
- Egg whites
- Nonfat/low-fat plain regular or Greek yogurt
- Nonfat/low-fat cottage cheese (low-sodium is best)
- Nonfat ricotta cheese

- Other nonfat cheeses
- Shrimp, scallops, and shellfish
  (avoid if you have high cholesterol)
- Tempeh
- Seitan
- Legumes

EAT UP TO FOUR TIMES PER WEEK

- Soy and tofu meals
- Tofu, firm
- Tofu, silken, firm (Mori-Nu)
- Edamame

EAT ONCE A WEEK

- Lean red meats (sirloin, tenderloin, beef loin, any loin cut)
- Fish: tuna or mackerel—only one of either per week

EAT ONLY ONCE PER MONTH

- Swordfish, shark, or tilefish
- Lean pork

In Chapter 11, I'll show you dozens of ways to get more of these low-fat, high-protein foods into your diet. For now, just remember that you can't go wrong with any of the choices under "Eat as Often as You Like," whether you're eating out or cooking for yourself.

Skinny Chick 10-Week Transformation

NAME: KATE B.

AGE: 27

TOTAL POUNDS LOST: 18

TOTAL INCHES LOST: 27.75

When I was younger, I was a gymnast, so I was always very muscular. As I got older, into high school, I wasn't involved in athletics and my eating habits were poor, so all of that bulk turned to fat.

I tried all the diets that everyone else has tried . . . but there was something so unforgiving about those diets that I could only make it through a couple of weeks. I would get off track and never felt I could get back on.

The Skinny Chicks program has so many positives. You feel great from the very beginning. Within a week, you feel a difference. Best of all, the program is forgiving. I needed a program that would help me to stay focused yet still live my life. During the course of the 10 weeks, I certainly found myself in a couple of situations where my food options were limited. In those cases, I would have whatever was being served, but I never felt that I was "cheating," and I never felt that I couldn't get right back on the program. I knew that my next meal was just 4 hours away, and I would get right back to eating a PC Combo.

When I walk out the door each morning, I take 60 seconds to go through what I'm going to be eating for the day, so there's a part of my life that's already planned out. I have control of that, and everything else falls into place from there.

It's really something when you're losing weight and you're eating right—the power that you feel to achieve more. Christine had us focus on our dreams and goals outside of health, and now I feel like everything's possible.

CHAPTER 8

The Carb Conspiracy

Carbohydrates are one of the most controversial subjects in the world of health and nutrition. It makes me angry when I hear people agree that you must reduce your carb intake to zero in order to lose weight. More than one celebrity client has stopped seeing me when I disagreed with this philosophy, and I have received ranting e-mails accusing me of being a pawn of the "greedy corporations" who are promoting carbohydrates for profit. When an idea gets into people's minds, whether it's right or wrong, it is sometimes very hard to shake it loose. And of course we all know someone who lost a great deal of weight on an extreme low-carb diet—only to gain it back almost immediately. Today the tide is turning, but slowly; for almost 30 years many thousands of people swallowed this concept hook, line, and sinker, and it's still part of today's nutritional landscape. Look in any grocery store and you can find a variety of products prominently labeled "low carb" or "no carb." Bookstores are still loaded with low-carb and no-carb recipe books. Despite the fact that only a few years earlier, before low-carb became the dietary buzzword du jour, the country had been swept away by the "low fat" diet fad and had managed to lose weight eating plenty of carbs, most people accepted the low-carb concept as gospel.

Many people, observing all the restaurant menus, books, and grocery store products, assume that the people behind these offerings, with all their money and resources, must have access to the best scientific research. How could all those people be wrong? Not only that, several scientific studies, like the one published in the *Journal of the American Medical Association* in 2007 that compared the Atkins diet (low-carbohydrate), the Zone diet (40/30/40), the Ornish diet (low-fat), and a low-fat/high-carb diet amongst a group of women, reported that the Atkins diet resulted in the most rapid weight loss.

So there you have it: inarguable evidence validated by scientific studies. And you know what?

They are absolutely right.

If you stop eating carbs right now and simply eat all the steak, bacon, chicken, sausage, pork, turkey, eggs, and dairy products you can find, you are going to lose weight—quickly. The science behind this is 100 percent accurate. Sounds great, right? So why aren't we all Skinny Minnies by now?

As I said before, nutrition is never quite that simple. There are, of course, more than a few problems with this approach:

- When you don't supply your body with glucose from outside sources, it will try to get the glucose it needs from the glycogen in liver tissue and from the muscles themselves.

- Too much protein may cause kidney stones and aggravate existing kidney problems.

- A low-carb diet can result in the loss of calcium. A Duke University study showed that urinary calcium losses rose significantly in individuals following a low-carbohydrate, high–animal protein diet for 6 months. If you are not getting enough calcium from milk or a calcium supplement, your body will start to take it from your own bones, making them very weak and brittle.

- Somewhere between 1 to 3 days into such a diet, when your body may enter ketosis (see "The Real Skinny on Ketosis"), you are truly breaking down fat for energy, but the breakdown is incomplete and there are several undesirable side effects.

- The worst problem, though, is not a matter of science but one of practical reality—most of us simply cannot stick to a low-carb

The Real Skinny on Ketosis

If you are familiar with the word *ketosis*, you have probably done some research into low-carb diets. Ketosis occurs when the body receives insufficient glucose during a fast or a low-carb diet. When glucose is not present, fat breakdown is incomplete and results in by-products known as ketone bodies. Your body is breaking down fat—but it is also breaking down muscle and other vital organs (this is, needless to say, a bad thing). Some of the undesirable side effects of ketosis include nausea, fatigue, bad breath, and dizziness, and even worse, abnormal heart rhythms, calcium depletion, and liver and kidney problems.

Many people don't know about these side effects and believe that ketosis is a fantastic way to lose body fat. In the mid-1990s, during the height of my fitness modeling days, I was one of those people. I remember buying "ketone strips" from the drugstore. These were white strips of treated paper you urinated on; if they changed color, that meant you had achieved ketosis. By the third day of limiting my carbs in order to achieve this state, I was half out of my mind, irrational, short-tempered, tired, and confused. Worst of all, I had no idea I was actually slowing my metabolism and breaking down muscle tissue. I am grateful every day that I now know the Skinny Chicks program is a much better way to lose fat!

diet. Ultimately, we cave in and binge on carbs to feed our starving bodies.

Speaking of reality, a closer look at the diet comparison study from *JAMA* reveals that few of the women actually stuck to their diets. Many on the non-Atkins diets were eating triple the amount of carbs they were supposed to eat. These women were in a scientific study conducted by top researchers at Stanford, a world-class university, and still they couldn't stick to their diets. What does that say for the rest of us? It says a lot.

When We Go on a Diet, Are We Really on a Diet?

The first thing we should all accept is that when we decide to go on a diet, the reality of what we eat is completely different from the diet we believe we are following. As you know from earlier chapters, I was just like the women in the *JAMA* study; I tried to keep from eating carbs, but the more I tried, the more my body would rebel and I would simply make up for the carb/energy deficit by overeating.

In fact, this was the subject of a segment I did for Rachael Ray's television show. In this segment, two women had 1 whole week of eating videotaped. All of their food choices were recreated for the show, and the entire week of meals for each of these two brave women was laid out on a table for all the world to see. As the camera panned down the table from one day to the next, you could make out the same pattern. There would be a few "dieting" days in a row, followed by a large binge day. After a binge day, most of us really starve ourselves—and these ladies were no different. But it was pretty shocking to see it laid out right before our eyes. And in reality, even on the days when they restricted their calories, there was always a cupcake, some cookies, a handful of animal crackers, a few glasses of wine, or some kind of treat that the women just "had to have." Their eating was never consistent, and it was never really a diet. It was the same with me, and it is the same with the majority of my clients.

So . . . if we don't really diet when we diet, what should we be doing? How can we lose weight? The key is to avoid dieting altogether. A diet represents restriction and deprivation. As a nutritionist, my job is to make you healthier, and to do that, I need you to eat real food and real meals—carbs and all.

Gotta Have Carbs

My experience reviewing thousands of food journals for my clients confirms what we all know in our hearts: Few of us can resist the urge to indulge in treats, most of them loaded with carbs. We live on Temptation Island, with carbs available everywhere, all the time. For some people, indulgence means a cookie here and there; for others it is a doughnut or two in the break room. For hard-core carbaholics like myself, it can mean eating an entire cake at one sitting. Your body will literally drag itself into the kitchen in the middle of the night to satisfy the carb urge. These urges are incredibly powerful.

When I read my clients' food journals, I can anticipate the carb binges. They usually take place after 2 or 3 days of limited carb consumption. After a few days of really small meals or protein-only meals, sure enough, the body makes up for the deficit as the person consumes a huge dinner followed by dessert, wine, and a late-night treat. The lack of stable blood sugar—the result of consuming too many or too few carbs—causes the erratic eating that results in fat storage.

Let's look at the facts for a moment:

1. Our cells need carbs for the glucose fuel to live.

2. We live in a world where there are irresistible carbs everywhere.

3. Even when we go on a diet and say we will avoid carbs, we are going to eat some—or a lot.

4. These binges are driven by the body's need for carbs (and the hormonal imbalance created by erratic blood sugar levels).

5. If we were to eat a steady flow of healthy carbs with a lean protein, we would not be struck by these urges to binge.

6. The only way to eat for weight loss and better health is to eat balanced meals including protein, carbs, and healthy fats every 4 hours.

I hope I have made my case.

Carbohydrates 101

The basic building blocks of carbohydrates are chains of sugar molecules. These sugar molecules are small enough to enter your bloodstream. By sugar molecules, I mean the same molecules that you sprinkle on your cornflakes. I know that bagels, pasta, and bread don't taste like table sugar, but they are all made up of the same basic molecules.

You may have heard that it is better to have "complex" rather than "simple" carbs. Simple carbs are small sugar molecules that are easily digested and absorbed through the intestines. Complex carbs are just simple sugar molecules linked together; your body has to break the chain into simple sugar molecules that can enter the bloodstream. Because of this extra step, digestion of complex carbohydrates takes longer, which gives you a steadier supply of energy that is less likely to be converted into fat and stored. Examples of simple carbs are sugar, fruit, honey, corn syrup, and maple syrup. Whole grains, potatoes, and vegetables are complex carbs. But really, the more important question is how quickly a carb enters the bloodstream, and it turns out that you can't tell that just by knowing whether a particular food is a simple or complex carbohydrate.

How the Glycemic Index Confuses the Issue

At one time it was thought that simple carbs were "bad" because they caused a spike in blood sugar, while complex carbs were "good" because they provided a steadier release of glucose that kept blood sugar stable. As it turns out, however, not all simple carbs are bad and not all complex carbs are good. In the 1980s, researchers developed what was thought to be a better way to identify the good from the bad. It's called the glycemic index (GI). Simply put, the glycemic index is a number given to carbs to reflect the rate at which they cause glucose levels in the blood to rise; the higher a carb's glycemic index rating, the faster it converts to glucose in the blood. Carbs with a GI of 55 or less cause only a tiny rise; those in the 55 to 70 range cause levels to rise a bit more; and carbs with GIs above 70 cause blood glucose levels to spike. For example, a baked potato has a GI level of 85 (big spike) and a sweet potato has a GI level of 54 (little blip); a pretzel has a GI of 83, while an apple has a GI of 36; and instant rice has a GI of 91, while brown rice has a GI of 55.

As you may already have guessed, high-GI carbs get the "bad" carb rap. Indeed, a meal that consists only of high-GI carbs will cause insulin levels to soar, pushing glucose into cells only to cause your blood sugar levels to fall lower than before you ate. You'll be hungry again and may find yourself at the snack machine pulling the lever for that bag of M&Ms. Meanwhile, that overload of insulin contributes to your weight gain by

The Real Skinny
on Eating by Numbers

It's not realistic to think you can live by assigning a number to every carb you eat. Bowl of strawberries: 32. Oatmeal cookie: 55. Melba toast: 70. Not to mention, those numbers can be deceiving: The GI of cornflakes is in the 80s, while a Snickers bar clocks in at 61! And carrots and watermelon both have off-the-chart GI readings; however, both are composed mostly of water and fiber and are chock full of nutrients—they actually contain only a very small amount of carbs. Going strictly by the numbers, you would miss out on those two healthy and delicious food choices.

Two of the worst offenders, according to the GI, are white rice and baked potatoes. Bear in mind, though, that these measurements are taken on the food in its pure state, with nothing added. Let me ask you this—have you ever eaten a bare baked potato in your whole lifetime? I think not. Putting butter on your baked potato will actually improve the GI (make it lower) because the fat in the butter basically introduces more traffic to the Blood Sugar Freeway and lowers the GI. Now don't think you can melt a whole stick of butter and a massive dollop of sour cream onto your baked potato; you don't want to put the fat content through the roof just to lower the GI. However, you can stuff that potato with some fat-free Cheddar cheese and broccoli . . . now we're talkin'!

stashing excess glucose into fat cells. And remember, high insulin levels also prevent fat cells from releasing stored energy when your body needs it. When you want to lose weight, you want those body fat storage cells to give up their stored energy; the more energy they pony up, the better your chances of successfully zipping up your "skinny" jeans. In contrast, a plate of low-GI carbs raises blood sugar slowly and steadily. Insulin levels rise only high enough to gently nudge glucose into waiting cells, where it is burned for energy, and your blood sugar stays steady for hours. Research shows that when your blood sugar is steady, you feel satisfied and full. That bag of M&Ms will stay in the vending machine to tempt another.

There are dozens of sites on the Internet and many books that will give you the GI value of any given food, should you wish to know. But, as with everything else we've been discussing, it isn't quite that simple. The GI is a measurement taken in a laboratory where the food is isolated. In real life, we almost always eat foods together with other foods. We hardly ever eat cereal without milk or rice without a main course. The best news is that when you eat a PC Combo, you lower the GI of any carb since the protein (and the healthy fats) will slow traffic on the Blood Sugar Freeway.

It's Not All about the Numbers

Here's how the GI can be deceiving. Doughnuts, jellybeans, cupcakes, Pop Tarts, Skittles, Fruit Loops, and Coca-Cola all have a lower GI than a plain baked potato, yet clearly none of these are healthy food choices. Chemically speaking, you could eat a grilled chicken breast with jellybeans and your body would be receiving the balance of protein and carbs that it needs to keep blood sugar stable. But this jellybean meal will not make you feel as full and healthy as the same grilled chicken breast eaten with a baked potato and fat-free sour cream. The jellybean feast is less substantial and not as wholesome, and you will simply not feel good after you eat it. If you've ever been a yo-yo dieter (and who hasn't?), you've experienced the difference in how your body feels after a healthy meal and after an unhealthy one. That feeling of well-being you get after a nutritious meal is crucial because without it, you will be much more tempted to grab that extra doughnut or drink that large blended coffee.

Use your common sense. If you're going to use the GI to choose foods, use it intelligently. For instance, natural sweeteners include sugar, honey, and agave nectar (a natural liquid sweetener extracted from the agave plant). Sugar has a GI of about 58; honey, because it comes from a variety of sources, can vary from about 32 to 80; and agave's GI is between 11 and 19. Several of the recipes in this book use agave nectar. That doesn't mean I never use honey—I especially like the taste of honey in my tea.

Any whole food (e.g., watermelon) is going to be a healthier choice than a food that is made of a variety of ingredients including chemical preservatives (e.g., ice cream or jellybeans). You don't want to overdo either of these foods, but watermelon (an excellent source of potassium, lycopene, and vitamins A, C, and B$_6$) will certainly leave you feeling healthier than ice cream. So don't just go down the GI list and choose a low number for your carbs. Instead, choose a healthy carbohydrate to eat with your lean protein at every meal.

The Perils of the Lonely Carb

The Harvard School of Public Health recommends whole grain cereals and breads, steel-cut oats, whole wheat pasta, and beans while discouraging potatoes. I completely agree that these are great healthy choices. But on the Skinny Chicks program, you have the option of eating potatoes, white rice, and pasta, should you want them, *as long as* they are accompanied by a lean protein and a healthy fat. Otherwise, you will definitely cause your blood sugar to rise and fall dramatically. Generally speaking, the best way to consume a carb is in a state as close to its natural, fresh-off-the-plant form as possible. The more you chop it, grind it, wash it, and bleach it, the less time it takes for your body to break it down into a simple sugar molecule. For instance, wheat starts out as a whole grain, is then stripped of its outer layer (where most of the nutrients live), and is eventually processed and bleached and filled with preservatives until we see it on the grocery store shelf as part of a loaf of white bread. A whole apple is digested more slowly than applesauce, which is digested more slowly than apple juice. All of these must always be combined with a lean, healthy protein at every meal to cause plenty of traffic on the Blood Sugar Freeway.

When you begin the Skinny Chicks' eating plan, you will only eat super-healthy carbs and PC Combos for the first 2 weeks. This gets your weight loss off to a nice, quick, healthy start. I call this phase, appropriately, the kick-start. Then, later, you will incorporate all your favorite carbs into your eating plan for life. This will give you the freedom to live and enjoy life without giving up your favorite foods (most of them, anyway).

Skinny Chick 10-Week Transformation

NAME: JEANNE M.

AGE: 53

TOTAL POUNDS LOST: 18

TOTAL INCHES LOST: 20.75

When I turned 40, I felt like I was cursed with the fat gene. The forties were all about the "F" words for me: fat, flabby, frumpy. I just kept putting on weight and I couldn't get it off. I tried everything to get my metabolism working again and even hired a personal trainer, but nothing was happening. I kept gaining weight and I was very frustrated—another "F" word. Then I found out about the Skinny Chicks program.

Now that I'm in my fifties, and I've been following the Skinny Chicks program, there are some more "F" words—but this time it's "fabulous." I feel "fantastic." I'm "firming" up, and I feel "faster" at everything I do.

Before I started the program, I had bad eating habits. I didn't know that I needed to combine carbohydrates with protein. I was one of those people who bought into the whole no-carb diet. I lost weight quickly, but it would come back on and it wouldn't come off again. When I started combining proteins with carbohydrates and eating four times a day as Christine advised me, I dropped a size in 3 weeks. Then I dropped another size after 6 weeks on the program. I have more weight to lose, but I am on the fast track to losing a lot more weight and getting back into shape.

CHAPTER 9

The Fat
Fear Factor

I once saw the late comedian Sam Kinison perform his stand-up routine. Near the end, he got all quiet and sensitive. In a soft, caring voice, he said, "You women, if there is something you want us men to do, any little things that we can do to make you happy . . . " He paused for a moment, then he hollered as only he could, "THEN WHY DON'T YOU GIVE US SOME POSSIBLE CLUE WHAT THE HECK IT IS???!!! TELL US!!!!! WE'LL DO IT!!!" It is hard to convey in writing how funny Sam was, but his point was this: Don't make me guess—just keep it simple. People losing weight have the same plea: Just tell me what not to eat. Fewer carbs? Fine. Less fats? No problem.

Before carbs were singled out as dietary villains, our country tried the "low-fat" approach. Soon dieters were chowing down guiltlessly on fat-free cookies, fat-free ice cream, and fat-free salad dressing. The theory was as simple as it gets: To *be* less fat, *eat* less fat.

So what happened? America got fatter and fatter, that's what happened. All those food manufacturers who jumped on the fat-free bandwagon forgot to remind us that fat free does not mean calorie free. And we consumers, thinking we had found the once-and-for-all, final-answer, easy way to lose weight, did not stop to read the labels of the foods we were buying.

We now know that we need fats just as we need carbs. We just don't need as many fats as most of us consume.

Fats are a hot political topic right now as we observe government bans on trans fats and constant media outcries about obesity. Skinny Chicks (a.k.a. healthy people) should understand what's up with fat, and what fat does on the inside of the body as well as the outside. Fats are an important subject, and this chapter will review and explain the various types and functions of fats, when they are appropriate, and why it's not a good idea to cut fats completely out of your diet repertoire.

Meet Joleen, Who Had No Idea

A few years ago I worked with a mother of three small children, who told me I came highly recommended by some of her fellow school moms. Joleen was whip-smart, well-educated, and very active chasing after her toddlers every day. Despite her activity level and some extreme dieting, she could not shed the baby weight from her third child. Joleen told me that losing her pregnancy weight after the first two children had been really easy because she would just restrict carbohydrates and exercise, and the weight would simply come off. But not this time around.

The first thing I asked Joleen to do was to keep a 24-hour food journal the day before our first consultation appointment, which is my usual procedure for new clients. When Joleen arrived at my office, I performed my standard tests: body fat analysis using digital skin fold calipers, body comp test (also to measure body fat) using bioelectrical impedance, girth measurements, and blood sugar analysis. I calculated her pounds of body fat versus lean tissue. Her body fat percentage was 28 percent. As a reference, anything over 25 percent for an adult woman is considered overweight, while 30 percent body fat is considered obese. Joleen was shocked because she was a size 8 and did not feel like she had high body fat. I explained to her that most women who come into my office start out at about 33 percent body fat, which made her body fat percentage actually lower than my average client. I went on to tell her that when I first began my nutrition certification program, I actually started out at 28 percent body fat myself, even though I was an avid exerciser and low-carb dieter at the time.

Next, I reviewed her food journal and immediately saw that for breakfast she was consuming 22 grams of fat, most of it saturated. She used one pat of butter (10 grams of fat) to fry her two eggs (8 grams of fat). For a midmorning snack she would consume two handfuls of nuts (30 grams of fat), and for lunch she would have a big salad (surprise!) with lots of meat, greens, and 4 to 6 tablespoons of ranch dressing (approximately 42 grams of fat). So, by lunchtime, this mother of three had consumed 84 grams of fat! That is twice my recommended fat intake for a full day. Her afternoon snack was either two whole-milk cheese cubes (15 grams of fat) or two handfuls of nuts (30 grams of fat). Finally, her dinner was grilled, roasted, or pan-fried meat and a side of steamed vegetables with one or two pats of butter. I informed her that her daily intake of fat was approximately 120 grams (I recommend around 40 grams per day). That is 1,080 calories from fat. Her daily caloric intake, including fat and protein, added up to 2,100 calories.

Joleen was shocked to realize how much fat she was consuming. Nor had she realized that it was mostly artery-clogging saturated fat. I told her she was not alone, and that many women were eating this way because they had experienced rapid weight loss during the first few weeks of low-carb diets. However, for most women there comes a time when the weight loss stops and the body decides enough is enough. That's where the Skinny Chicks program comes in.

I explained to Joleen that she *should* eat fat, and that fat is good for her, but that to lose weight, most women need to eat no more than 10 to 13 grams of fat per meal (even less if you have a small frame). I had her incorporate healthy, high-fiber carbohydrates, lean proteins, and healthy fats into each meal. After only 1 week on my program, she came into my office and I weighed her. She had lost 4 pounds—a good week. But I knew that Joleen, who had been such a die-hard low-carb advocate, might have a hard time taking my advice about eating a balance of protein, carbs, and fats. Often, low-carb advocates pay me for my advice but then they simply go on a super-strict zero-carb diet. So I didn't want to get too excited until I did her body fat test. If she'd lost 4 pounds of muscle, it would mean she'd restricted carbs (restricting carbs for a week will cause the body to burn lots of muscle tissue). But if the 4 pounds she had lost were from body fat, I would know that she had cut back on fat intake and added in some healthy carbs. I did her body fat test and, sure enough, she was down 1 percent body fat, which means that she lost 4 pounds of fat in only 1 week! Joleen was delighted to be losing body fat and losing it from her waist first. With these quick results, she continued on my program and lost all of her extra baby weight in 6 weeks, for a total weight loss of 12 pounds of fat. She is now back to the weight and size she was on her wedding day. To this day, she comes to my office every 4 months just to check in and have me test her body fat. Joleen is so excited about what she learned on my program that I receive referrals from her constantly. (I call them the Pacific Palisades Skinny Moms Club!) They are all very successful on my program, and I believe that moms are some of my most special clients because they are passing down their nutrition habits to their precious little ones . . . the children.

Fast Fat Facts

The reality is that for weight loss, it still is and always will be important to reduce excess dietary fat intake. Why? Because fat in your food can translate into fat on your tummy, buns, thighs, arms, or anywhere your body fat tends to accumulate. Here is how it happens: Of the three energy-yielding nutrients (proteins, carbohydrates, and fats), fats contain the most energy/calories per gram. By now you probably know that both protein and carbohydrates have 4 calories per gram, while fat has 9 calories per gram. When we eat too much, it doesn't matter what we are eating, our bodies can and will convert it to fat storage. But the metabolic pathway from dietary fat to body fat requires the fewest steps when compared with carbohydrate and protein breakdown. Fat goes from lips to hips more easily than any other nutrient. This is one of the reasons I recommend limiting daily fat intake to 20 percent of your overall caloric intake. Too much of a good thing is never good . . . right?

For many of my clients, the whole low-fat-no-fat fiasco has caused a great deal of confusion and frustration. It's important to clear up this misunderstanding; in fact, it's a matter of life and death. So here goes:

All bodily cells need fats to function. Fats provide fuel for cells. They also provide raw materials for building cell membranes and the outer layer that surrounds the cell and controls what goes in and out of the cell itself. Fats also create protective sheaths that surround nerves. Fats are the building blocks for some hormones as well as for chemicals that control muscle contractions and blood clotting. The body can make most of the fats it needs from any fat in the diet or from carbohydrates. However, there are a small number of fats your body needs that cannot be created within the body. These are called essential fats, and they only come from the foods we eat. That's why it's not only unnecessary to avoid fat in your diet, it's vital that you include it. However, just as with carbs, all fats are not created equal. In total, there are four kinds of fat: one you should make an effort not to overdo, one you should avoid like the plague, and two that are must-haves.

The "Bad" Fats

- **Saturated fats:** These are generally solid at room temperature and come mainly from animals and animal products such as whole milk, cream, butter, cheese, red meat, and palm oil. Why are these fats bad for you? To begin with, saturated fats cause LDL ("bad") levels of cholesterol to rise, because they prevent cholesterol from getting inside the cells. (Cholesterol is not all bad—it is required for the formation of bile acids, which are needed for fat digestion; it is used to make important hormones such as estrogen and progesterone; and it is involved in the formation of vitamin D in the skin.) That leaves excess cholesterol floating around in the bloodstream, where it can become part of the plaque that builds up in your arteries. According to the American Heart Association (AHA), one American dies every 35 seconds of a heart-related disease. The number one suspect in heart disease is saturated fat.

  However, here is something you must understand. Saturated fats have their good points. They are a good source of energy when our bodies are low on fuel; they act as "shock absorbers" for our internal organs; and they insulate us from the cold. Saturated fats are only harmful when they're consumed in excess. One little pat of butter will not do you in—but great gobs of it on a stack of pancakes every Sunday will probably clog your arteries. The AHA recommends choosing fats and oils with 2 grams or fewer of saturated fat per tablespoon.

- **Trans fats:** Trans fat is vegetable oil that has been heated in the presence of hydrogen gas and nickel oxide, in a process known as partial hydrogenation. That transforms vegetable oil into solid fat. This explains how we get margarine and Crisco, which was introduced to the public in 1911. In 1984, fast-food restaurants stopped using beef fat for frying and switched to partially hydrogenated vegetable oil (a.k.a. trans fats) because it was less expensive and it prolonged the shelf life of the food. Ironically, the development of trans fats came at the urging of consumer groups who wanted restaurants to find a substitute for the saturated fats they had been using. By 2002, an FDA advisory panel realized that trans fats were more harmful than saturated fats, and the Institute of Medicine concluded that the safest amount of trans fats for humans is zero. So why is the food industry still allowed to use trans fats? I don't really know. My guess is that it won't be allowed for much longer.

    Manufacturers love trans fats because they extend the shelf life of food, but too much trans fat in your diet will cut *your* shelf life short. Trans fat is worse for you than saturated fat; it can raise bad LDL cholesterol and lower good HDL cholesterol and has been linked to both heart disease and diabetes. Putting trans fats into your body is like dropping grains of sand into a Swiss watch; sooner or later, it will stop working. Trans fats will cause arteries to clog up and eventually contribute to heart attacks and strokes, so it is a good idea to find foods that are cooked without them. They are so harmful that New York City, in a move that made history, banned trans fats from all city restaurants. You can avoid trans fats by staying away from fast foods and by reading the labels of packaged goods. Anything that contains hydrogenated oil or partially hydrogenated oil should be put back unopened where it can sit and live out its shelf life alone and untouched. And don't be fooled by "diet" foods like protein bars and fat-free ice cream; they may contain trans fats as well.

The "Good" Fats

- **Monounsaturated fats:** These fats are liquid at room temperature, but start to solidify at refrigerator temperature. They come from certain plant oils, including olive, canola, and peanut oils, as well as avocado. Eat up!

- **Polyunsaturated fats:** These fats are liquid at room temperature and in the fridge. You'll find polyunsaturated fats in seeds and in oils made from corn, soybeans, sesame, safflower, and sunflower, as well as in nuts and fish. Replacing the saturated fats in your diet with unsaturated fats may help lower your blood cholesterol level. However, before you go out and chow down on fat (unsaturated or otherwise), remember this: Fat contains more than twice the calories of either protein or carbohydrate. You only need a small amount—10–15 grams—of healthy fat in every meal, always eaten as part of a PC Combo, of course.

The "Superhero" Fats

If you're looking for the fats your body needs to save the day (as far as your health is concerned), you'll call on the superhero of the fat world: omega-3s.

Both omega-3s and omega-6s are essential fatty acids (EFAs), necessary for human health. Our bodies can't produce EFAs, so we must get them from the foods we eat. Omega-3 is typically found in fish, flaxseed, and walnuts. Omega-6 is found in corn, soy, canola, safflower, and sunflower oil. A balance of these two fats is necessary for optimal health. Unfortunately, most Americans consume a far larger number of omega-6s than omega-3s, and this is a problem, as an excess of omega-6 can cause serious health problems. That means you should try to consume less vegetable oils and meat, and more fish and fish oil.

There are three kinds of omega-3 fatty acids. The first two are eicosa-pentaenoic acid (EPA) and docosahexaenoic acid (DHA). Also known as fish oils, these omega-3s are found mostly in coldwater fish, including salmon, trout, white tuna, king mackerel, sea bass, herring, oysters, and sardines. The third omega-3 is alpha-linolenic acid (ALA) and comes from plant sources including flaxseed, walnuts, sunflower seeds, canola oils, soy, wheat germ, and dark leafy greens. Some of the many benefits of omega-3s include:

- **Weight loss.** EFAs help improve insulin sensitivity, help prevent type 2 diabetes, and help keep your blood sugar stable, which, as we know, is essential for weight loss and maintenance. Fats in the bloodstream help slow down the speed at which glucose flows. EFAs also increase your body's metabolic rate and help burn fat. Does this mean you can eat a ton of fat with your carbs? No; not if you want to have a fit and lean body. Think of fats as a small flavorful helper, but not your primary fuel.

  One interesting study from the University of South Australia showed that women who ate fish or took fish oil supplements and exercised lost more weight than those who did either one alone. The study's researchers believe that the fatty acids in fish oils activate enzymes that enhance the fat-burning effects of exercise.

- **Heart health.** Omega-3s are polyunsaturated, so they don't cause plaque buildup in the arteries that can lead to heart disease. A 2006 study from Harvard University determined that 250 milli-grams a day of DHA and EPA from fish or fish oil supplements helped reduce the risk of dying from a heart attack by 36 percent.

- **Joint health.** Omega-3s have been shown to decrease the produc-tion of inflammatory proteins called cytokines, which are known to play a role in stripping cartilage and eroding bone. And studies have shown that people who consume fish oils have fewer tender joints and decreased stiffness.

- **Mood lifter.** The National Institutes of Health has stated that two 4-ounce servings of fatty fish, such as salmon, halibut, or canned light tuna, per week can significantly raise your levels of serotonin, a mood-boosting brain chemical. Other studies have shown that people who live in countries with higher rates of fish consumption have lower rates of clinical depression, bipolar disorder, and postpartum depression. Not only that, people who consumed higher levels of EPA and DHA were less likely to report feeling "blue." Bill Sears, MD, associate clinical professor of pediatrics at the University of California, Irvine School of Medicine, told the *Los Angeles Times* in May 2008, "There's a lot of good science on food and the brain, particularly in the area of omega-3 fatty acids. In fact, the first so-called medicine I prescribe for a child with any type of learning, behavior, or mood disorder is high doses of omega-3."

● **Cognitive improvement.** Your mother was right; fish is brain food. EFAs are essential to brain health. The brain is made up of 60 percent fat. Diets that are too low in fat can have serious cognitive consequences. On the other hand, studies have shown that people who eat fish two or three times per week are half as likely to experience age-related cognitive decline, including Alzheimer's disease.

● **Great skin and shiny hair.** You can often tell a person who is deficient in fatty acids because they will have dry, flaky skin, dandruff, and eczema. EFAs help your skin maintain its elasticity and youthful glow, and they help keep hair healthy and shiny.

I recommend that everyone eat fish three times per week to get your requirement of omega-3 fats. If you are not able to do that, you need to take an omega-3 supplement for the many benefits. Simply O-3 is the name of my omega-3 supplement—you can find it at www.christineavanti.com.

Nuts about Nuts

Many experts recommend a handful of nuts if you are hungry, because, they say, nuts are a great source of protein. However, I teach my clients to think of nuts as a "good fat" and not a protein. If you look at the nutrition facts for nuts, you will see that nuts are much higher in fat than in protein. And considering the fact that fat in our foods converts into fat

The Real Skinny on ALA

Alpha-linolenic acid (ALA) is a type of plant-derived omega-3 fatty acid that has many of its own benefits. It has been shown to reduce the risk of total cholesterol, lower LDL (bad) cholesterol, help lower blood pressure, and keep platelets from becoming sticky, thus reducing the risk of a heart attack. A 16-year study from Harvard University of nearly 77,000 female nurses found that women with the highest intake of ALA (1.5 grams per day) had a 46 percent lower risk of sudden cardiac death than those who consumed only 0.7 gram per day. I find the easiest way to ensure that I'm getting my fair share of ALA is to sprinkle some ground flaxseed on top of my cereal or oatmeal in the morning or on my yogurt parfait afternoon meals, or to add it to delicious fruit smoothies.

on our bodies, I cannot tell clients to use nuts as a protein source if they need to lose weight. If you are at your optimal weight and your metabolism is healthy, by all means ignore me and go nuts! But for myself and everyone on the Skinny Chicks program, I say consider nuts a "good fat."

Many diets also recommend nut butters, such as peanut butter, almond butter, and macadamia butter. But these are also inadequate protein sources. I constantly see new clients in my office who truly believe that by spreading peanut butter on their morning bagel, they are getting a ton of protein. Sadly, they are getting a double dose of fat (healthy fat but still fat) and a single dose of an incomplete protein (non–animal based proteins oftentimes do not offer all nine essential amino acids; thus they are called incomplete proteins). Spreading peanut butter on a whole wheat bagel would technically give you a complete protein, but you're still getting a double dose of fat.

Read the chart on the opposite page, and look closely at the grams of protein and grams of fat in each; you will notice there is about twice as much fat as there is protein in most types of nuts and nut butters.

FOOD	SERVING SIZE	PROTEIN (G)	FAT (G)
Almonds	2 oz	12.5	30
Almond butter	2 Tbsp	5	18
Brazil nuts	2 oz	8	38
Cashews	2 oz	9	26
Cashew butter	2 Tbsp	5	14
Hazelnuts	2 oz	8	34
Macadamia nuts	2 oz	4	43
Peanuts	2 oz	13	28
Peanut butter	2 Tbsp	7	16
Pecans	2 oz	5	42
Pine nuts	2 oz	8	39
Pistachios	2 oz	12	26
Sunflower seeds	2 oz	11	20
Walnuts	2 oz	14	33

Here are the exceptions:

Soy nuts	2 oz	21	13
Soy nut butter	2 Tbsp	7	11

Perhaps even more importantly, neither a handful of nuts nor a few tablespoons of nut butter will satisfy your hunger the way a serving of the lean proteins beginning on page 287 will. I have clients who are in tears because they are so tired of being hungry. A handful of nuts is not enough, and they wind up overeating later in the day to make up for it. So stop driving yourself nuts with the notion that nuts will facilitate weight loss, because they seldom do.

Skinny Chick 10-Week Transformation

NAME: JENNIFER H.

AGE: 46

TOTAL POUNDS LOST: 14

TOTAL INCHES LOST: 25.5

I was one of those people who was always very skinny. Even when I gained weight, I felt that I was skinny. But when I got into my forties and was going through premenopause, I put on about 20 pounds. For the past 10 years, I've gone on many different diets, and I would lose 5 or 10 pounds, but I'd never feel good about it and would always gain it right back.

With Christine's Skinny Chicks program, there were two really cool things. I had accumulated this belly fat, which I absolutely hated. Her program is the first one of all the nutrition plans where the belly fat came off first. In addition, I lost weight in my legs, and that feels great, too. You're not just losing weight on the scale, you're also losing inches. And your body shape changes. It's amazing. Even my clothes from when I was thinner don't fit anymore because the whole body changes on the Skinny Chicks program. You really lengthen everything, and you get strong and lean and you lose all that excess fat.

What surprised me were the other benefits I got from the program. I've suffered from migraine headaches my whole life. In recent years, I've been taking a prescription medicine plus Tylenol all the time. I was at the point where I was getting four to six migraines a month. I have two teenagers, I own a business, and I just don't have time for that kind of illness. However, since the second week of the Skinny Chicks program, I haven't had one migraine. I think that is just a miracle.

I grew up in the fast-food generation. We're all busy and on the go all the time. But what I've learned is that even on the go, you can eat healthfully. I learned not to let myself get to the point where I'm starving, to eat combinations of carbs and proteins, and to make sure I'm not eating a lot of processed foods. As Christine says, if you can't read it, you probably shouldn't eat it.

I have two teenage girls, and it's very important to me that they don't see me on some fad diet because I want to set a good example for them. On the Skinny Chicks program, we all tend to eat healthy meals together.

This program has made me realize that no matter what point you're at in your life, you can still always learn something and get remotivated. I feel great, I look great, and it permeates into other parts of my life.

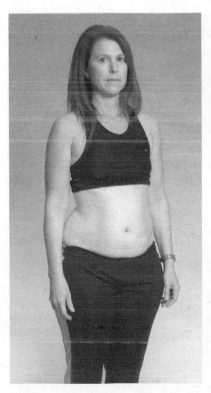 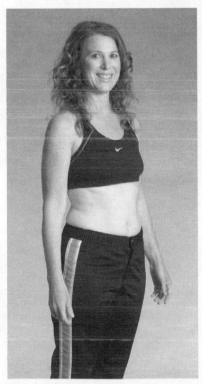

Skinny Chick Chat

Dear Christine: One of the reasons I never succeed on a diet is that I'm usually hungry all the time. This makes me crazy (just ask my friends and family). What can I do to lose weight without being hungry all day?

ROSEMARY T., CLEVELAND

Rosemary: That is one of the greatest things about my program. Rather than depriving yourself, you get to eat real meals every 4 hours. Since you are eating this often and the meals are a balance of protein, carbs, and some healthy fats, you won't feel hungry until it is time for your next meal. Remember—try to keep healthy fats down to 10 grams of fat per meal and eat them with the rest of your meal, rather than alone as you would a handful of nuts. I think you will be much more satisfied and happier.

EAT WELL, CHRISTINE

CHAPTER 10

Drink Yourself Skinny

When I was a teenager, one of my first jobs was at Baskin-Robbins. (Hey, I needed some way to pay for my Duran Duran albums.) But Baskin-Robbins has recently distinguished itself in nutrition infamy. In March of 2008, *Men's Health* magazine ranked the Baskin-Robbins large Heath Bar Shake as the "unhealthiest drink in America," no small achievement. At 2,310 calories and 108 grams of fat (64 of them "bad" saturated fats), this drink is destined to take up permanent residence on your buns and around your middle. It weighs in at 6 times my recommended caloric intake for a single meal and 11 times the fat. If you ate an otherwise balanced diet, but drank one of these each day, you could go from skinny to fat in a few weeks with no effort. The only people who should ever drink these are actors trying to bulk up to play overweight characters, which is a world market of about 10 people. (Even for them, I would recommend something without so much saturated fat.) Sorry, Baskin-Robbins—I appreciate your giving me the job when I needed it, but I can't recommend your shake.

Our country is awash in delicious but horrifically unhealthy drinks. In 2007, a panel of experts on nutrition and health estimated that about 21 percent of calories consumed by Americans over the age of 2 come from beverages, especially soft drinks and fruit drinks with added sugar. Compounding the problem, the panel found, is that beverages have "weak satiety properties"—they don't fill you up or curb your appetite—and people do not compensate for the beverage calories by eating less food.

Every time you pull into a drive-thru, a Starbucks, a convenience store, or a grocery store, you encounter irresistible blended beverages. You might decide to stop at Jamba Juice, for instance. Juice is good for you, right? Well, it may not be as bad as the Baskin-Robbins Heath Bar Shake, but one 32-ounce Peanut Butter Moo'd contains more than 1,100 calories, 30 grams of fat, and 199 grams of carbs. What about frappuccinos? Easily 600 calories. Only one-quarter of the calories of the Heath Bar Shake, but still far from my target number. Remember, you want to keep each of your entire meals around 400 calories and under 10 grams of fat.

Even flavored waters aren't "free" food. They taste great and provide vitamins, right? Well, maybe so, but they also contain about 120 calories per bottle—still more than you should be taking in between meals. Look at it this way: If you drink two "healthy" Vitamin Waters per day in addition to your usual calorie intake, you could gain 1 pound in 14.5 days!

Okay, so what number is low enough? What is the right number of calories in a drink?

Zilch. Nada. Zero. Not one. If you want to slim down, you should not be getting a single calorie from your drinks.

What you should be drinking is water. Every doctor, every diet, and every nutrition plan says you need to drink at least 8 glasses of water every day. I agree—your body needs a lot of fresh water every day. What's confusing us now are the hundreds of varieties of water or "water-type" beverages available in every supermarket and convenience store in America.

It's extremely important to make the distinction between a sugary drink and water. You might look at a bottle and figure, "Hey, I know I need 8 glasses of water per day; why not make it a great-tasting drink? This drink is mostly water, but better tasting, and the label says it includes a bunch of vitamins (or antioxidants or other 'health benefits')." So instead of drinking water, you might choose to sip on a sweet drink all day long. When you do this every day, it really adds up. So before you buy that "healthy" watery drink, be sure to read the label to see what you're really getting.

What about Juice?

Most everybody knows by now that all the sugar and harmful ingredients in a soda are not going to help you lose weight. But what about fruit
juices? Aren't they a good source of vitamins, minerals, and phytonutri-
ents? Yes, they are, but they are also loaded with sugar in the form of
fructose. Drinking even natural fruit juices between meals is simply
pouring sugar into your bloodstream. As we learned, this can lead to
storage of body fat. However, having a small glass of juice with a meal is
fine as long as you recognize the juice as part of your carbohydrate portion. But for best results, I recommend you stick to zero-calorie beverages during your weight loss phase unless otherwise specified in the
Skinny Chicks' meal plan.

What happens if you drink fruit juice (or any other sugary drink) all
day long? Remember the fuel tanks we learned about in Chapter 3? If
you're drinking sugar all day, Tank 1 (blood sugar) will always be full
and you will never reach Tank 2 (glycogen in the liver and muscle tissue
plus body fat), and thus you'll never burn any body fat.

Now let's look at the caloric cost of drinking juice instead of water
with meals. One medium-size glass of orange juice contains about 150
calories. Suppose you started drinking one glass each day with breakfast
and did nothing else differently. In the course of a year, you would gain
about 16 pounds, but you wouldn't feel any more satiated because juice

is just liquid. If you simply swapped that glass of juice for water, you would theoretically lose 16 pounds in a year without feeling any hungrier or expending any additional effort.

However, there is a big difference between theory and reality. Yes, your body can get the water it needs either way, but the orange juice contains a lot of energy in the form of sugar. If you cut that out, your body will subconsciously reach for a few more bites to compensate for the lost energy of the orange juice. This might come in the form of a bag of potato chips or an extra scoop of rice, or maybe a few bites more of dessert at night. In theory, you simply change the juice for water, but in reality your body compensates.

So does that mean that all hope is lost? Of course not. Here is the plan:

1. Drink ice water all day long between meals to keep your body hydrated (I highly recommend you add some lemon slices to your ice water for the added flavor, the spalike feel, and the anti-oxidant benefits).

2. If you want to drink fruit juices, have them with meals and be sure to keep the overall amounts of protein, carbs, and healthy fats in balance.

3. In moderation (no more than two or three times per week), you can drink a diet soda or another zero-calorie drink.

It is as simple as that.

Coffee Breaks: I'll Take a Direct Injection, Please

Everybody needs to take a coffee break now and then, and I don't have a real issue with coffee or even caffeine. Caffeine, when taken to excess, can interfere with the function of the adrenal system and the nervous system. But research studies have shown that a single cup of coffee each day will not harm you and can increase clarity of mind and alertness (thank goodness).

The problem is that you don't go to the espresso bar for regular drip.

You want something creamy, dreamy, and delicious. I strongly believe that the innovation of high-calorie beverages, including coffee drinks, is a major cause of America's increasing obesity rates. Most patrons of these coffee joints are ordering lattes, caramel macchiatos, and frappuccinos—all of which are very high in calories and fats. To make matters worse, many people add a huge dollop of whipped cream on top.

A venti frappuccino with whipped cream packs almost 600 calories—almost 50 percent more than I recommend for a full meal. But a frappuccino is definitely *not* a meal. It briefly postpones your appetite for lunch or dinner, but it doesn't fill you up or satisfy you.

This doesn't mean you need to steer clear of Starbucks altogether. There are several great zero-calorie drinks that you can order at your favorite coffee spot. The very best order, hands down, is green tea. Green tea is a natural fat burner due to its thermogenic properties, which enhance fatty acid oxidation. Green tea is also loaded with antioxidants called catechins that are thought to help with weight loss. In one study, metabolic rate was increased by an average of 266 calories per day, which means you could lose approximately 1 pound every 2 weeks simply by drinking 8 to 10 cups of tea (or by taking a 90-milligram green tea extract supplement). Green tea also has an amino acid in it called L-theanine, which boosts alpha brain waves and promotes alert relaxation, and who doesn't need a little of that each day? In addition to its weight loss and cognitive benefits, tea contains anticancer agents and reduces the risk of heart disease, hypertension, tooth decay, and even bad breath. With all the wonderful benefits of tea, I highly recommend that you get into the habit of ordering green tea (or any tea—white, green, oolong, or black) during your daily coffee run.

If you can't make the transition to tea, the next best things to order are espressos, Americanos, and regular drip coffees. All are nearly calorie-free and won't interfere with your metabolism or appetite. As soon as you start adding milk to your drink, even fat-free milk, you are consuming calories, altering your meal schedule, and keeping your body from dipping into Tank 2 (always burning blood sugar for fuel, never getting to body fat). For that reason, if you *must* have a latte, mocha, or macchiato, order them with

Skinny Chick 10-Week Transformation

NAME: JOY L.

AGE: 48

TOTAL POUNDS LOST: 14

TOTAL INCHES LOST: 19.25

When I was young, my best friend and I were called Fat and Skinny. She was the fat one and I was the skinny one. We'd sit on the front porch and I would eat a whole bag of Doritos, a whole bag of Double Stuf Oreos, and a diet soda. I could eat anything I wanted, and I never exercised. I never watched my weight because I never had to.

When I was pregnant with my first baby, I actually gained 85 pounds and then lost it all. During my second pregnancy, I gained about the same, and I lost almost all of it except for maybe 5 pounds. I probably weighed about 110. I stayed there for years and years. Then it started to creep up, and when I was 35, I weighed about 115. I stayed there until about 42. Then I had a hysterectomy, so I went through menopause, and I packed on about 20 pounds overnight. I started to exercise—I would run and work out, and I still ended up gaining weight.

Over the years, I've had several trainers and nutritionists. My first trainer had me drink a lot of shakes. When you're drinking shakes and eating maybe one meal, you're going to lose the weight. I lost about 20 pounds, and of course, I gained it right back. Then I went to another nutritionist, and I lost weight with her, too. But she limited me from having a lot of foods that I enjoy. The Skinny Chicks program is very different from any of the other things I've tried. All women think we'll lose weight eating salads. Obviously, it's not true because most of the people who are eating salads are not thin. But they keep ordering salads.

I love eating all the foods we're allowed to eat. I didn't eat a lot of carbs before. I would only have them once in a while. Now I can have a carb at every meal, and I'm losing weight!

Losing weight makes me feel like myself again. Some people said I didn't need to lose weight. But it's not about what anybody else thinks; it's about what you *feel*. I felt horrible and I didn't want to go out or meet anybody because when you don't feel good about yourself, you're not going to feel good about anything.

It's really hard when you're going through menopause, and just getting older in general, to lose weight and then keep it off. But this is working. The program has definitely taught me a lot about nutrition and what happens to your body if you don't eat right and you eat a lot of sugar, or if you eat only carbs or only protein, which is what I was doing. What a change this program has made in my life. I plan on eating this way forever.

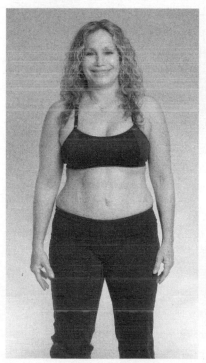 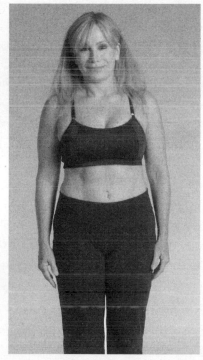

fat-free milk, order the smallest size, and drink them only along with a meal. Again, keep track of the total nutrient amounts and balances. And if you must have a frappuccino, choose a tall Starbucks frappuccino light, espresso-flavored with no whip. It has only 80 calories and 5 grams of fat. Heck, go ahead and make it a double, if you really must!

If You're Boozin', You Aren't Losin'

Let's face it. We all love to party after a hard day at the office, to celebrate a special occasion, or just as a release of the tensions of everyday life. And for many of us, it's just not a party if there is no alcohol. However, if you really want to lose weight, you should bone up on your alcohol facts.

Drinking alcohol makes it much harder to lose body fat.

The problem with alcohol is that it goes right to the front of the line in the liver, like the person who marches right up to the counter at the DMV when you've been waiting in line for an hour. Rude! The liver normally prefers to break down proteins, carbs, and most importantly fatty acids, but when pushy alcohol is present, all the nice little nutrients have to go to the end of the line. Alcohol also permanently changes the structure of liver cells, which impairs the liver's ability to metabolize fats. So alcohol generally slows down weight loss. And of course, when you are tipsy or drunk, you are more likely to grab whatever you see and eat it. That doesn't help us fit into our little red dresses, now does it?

If you are truly to lose weight, you must avoid all forms of alcohol as much as possible. Regardless of alcohol's "benefits," it still slows down the metabolism of fatty acids within the liver and makes it more difficult to lose weight. While you're trying to lose weight, definitely avoid mixed drinks and hard alcohol. Sorry! No more chocolate martinis, raspberry mojitos, or blended margaritas. They are extremely high in calories.

So what is my advice? I say go out and buy yourself the most expensive bottle of red wine you can afford. Then, when you want to enjoy some, pour yourself a half-glass and enjoy that baby like it is the finest beverage on Earth. You know you would rather have a quarter-glass of Opus than a whole bottle of 2 Buck Chuck, and when it is that expensive, you definitely won't drink too much. Red wine contains antioxi-

The Real Skinny on Beer Bellies

Some people believe that beer causes beer bellies because of the maltose (sugar) content in beer. The logic is that wine won't make you fat, but beer will because it is made of maltose. That would be correct if only it were that simple. Maltose is very high on the GI list—but beer is not pure maltose. Most beers contain only trace amounts of maltose since it is mostly fermented into alcohol. It's calories that cause beer bellies. Plenty of men who have never had a drop of beer have beer bellies, and indeed the term *beer belly* itself is a misnomer.

dants and resveratrol—a compound that has been observed to have an anti-clotting effect in the blood (believed to reduce the risk of heart attacks and strokes). A small glass (about 2 ounces) has about 40 calories and will not slow down your weight loss. A standard-size serving of wine is about 5 ounces, and some wine glasses hold much more than that—so it pays to measure the amount of wine you're drinking.

Here are some examples for you. These calorie counts are approximate, as every bartender has his or her own recipe and the calories vary according to ingredients and portions. But to give you a general idea:

COCKTAIL	CALORIES
Long Island Iced Tea	780
Frozen margarita	740
Margarita	490
Piña colada	460
Mai tai	350
Sangria	310
Martini	160–175
Mojito	150–220

Does that mean you can never have a mixed drink? Of course not! Make it yourself and make room for it in your nutrition plan.

PART III

SKINNY CHICKS

PUT IT ALL

TOGETHER

CHAPTER 11

Skinny Chicks'
Meal Plans

Now that you have the lowdown on why it's important to keep your blood sugar at a steady level and how the mighty PC Combo is the key to success, it's time to put all this great newfound knowledge into action. That's where my meal plans come in, and you'll find a week's worth of kick-start meals and 2 weeks of everyday meals in the pages that follow to get you up and running.

But don't stop there. The Skinny Chicks program is designed to help you drop weight—serious amounts of weight—whether or not you incorporate exercise into your routine. But for optimal results and even greater, faster weight loss, I always recommend that my clients incorporate physical activity into their programs as well as nutritional supplements. This section will give you guidelines for beginner, intermediate, and advanced workouts to complement your meal plans as well as recommendations for safeguarding your health and well-being with dietary supplements.

If you're not currently exercising, I recommend you start with the beginner workout described on page 181 when you begin the kick-start program. Once you gain strength and endurance, you can graduate to one of the more advanced workouts. If you already work out on a regular basis, start with the intermediate or advanced workouts.

About the Meal Plans

Kick-start meals have approximately the same caloric value as the every-day meals, but are comprised of foods (particularly carbs) in their most natural, minimally processed states. You will see that only unprocessed foods are called for; no bread, pasta, cereals, or crackers. You'll still be eating a healthy balance of carbs and proteins, but the carbs are whole grains, fruits, and vegetables. I also recommend that you avoid restaurants and alcohol during this period. After 1 week, you can reintroduce some of the foods you've eliminated and enjoy an occasional meal out or a glass of wine.

While I have provided recipes for 1 full week of kick-start meals and 2 weeks' worth of everyday Skinny Chicks' meals, I recognize that not everyone has time to cook even once or twice, much less four times every day. If that's true for you, don't worry! Many of these meals are choices you can find readily on restaurant menus or that you can replace with a frozen entrée (just be sure to choose one that has the proper ratio of carbs to protein; see page 162 for an example). One trick I use all the time is dividing my restaurant meal, eating half and saving the rest for a quick, premade meal the next day. Not only is this a time saver, it makes nutritional sense, too, given how restaurant portions have bal-looned in recent years.

And if you really don't have time to cook at all, just choose a combina-tion of foods from the kick-start or everyday food lists from the Appendix on page 286, keeping the total calories at or below 400 and again main-taining the proper ratio of carbs to protein.

Lastly, remember that all of these recipes, as well as those starting on page 235, can be used interchangeably. In that section you'll find all the recipes referred to in the kick-start and the everyday weight loss plan, plus additional recipes that adhere to the Skinny Chicks' guidelines to be used as the cornerstones of your own meal plans as you work toward meeting your individual weight loss goal. As you've seen from the testimonials throughout this book, you can achieve remarkable results in just 10 weeks. Best of all, it's a way of eating you can really stick with. I should know; I've been doing it for 10 years and have enjoyed every minute of it.

The Skinny Chicks' Kick-Start 7-Day Plan

Why a kick-start plan? The best way to start real-life weight loss is to clear out your internal system so that your body can begin to release stored body fat. When your body is loaded with toxins, it responds by retaining water in an effort to dilute water-soluble toxins. Your body also retains fat in an effort to dilute fat-soluble toxins. Until you clear your body of these toxins, it will work overtime to store water and fat to protect itself and dilute these toxins. In addition to clearing out toxins, the kick-start program will help to stabilize blood sugar levels within the first few days. This is not a carbohydrate-restrictive program; rather, you will be eating a PC Combo at every meal. However, the carbohydrate choices are all natural, nonprocessed fresh fruits, vegetables, and whole grains. **Please note: The kick-start plan is a strict nutrition program and is only intended for short-term use.**

Benefits of the Kick-Start

1. You will drop 2 to 7 pounds or more of water, toxins, and possibly body fat within 7 days.

2. As you lose weight, your body releases toxins from fat cells into the bloodstream, which can be harmful. Detoxification can help bind up these harmful toxins and move them out of the body safely.

3. If you have a large amount of body fat to lose and you hit a plateau at any point on the Skinny Chicks program, it could be a result of too many toxins in your bloodstream. Coming back to the kick-start will likely break the plateau and get your fat burning going again.

Kick-Start Guidelines

- Eat a PC Combo every 4 hours.

- Can't eat every 4 hours? Simply cut the meal portions in half and eat every 2 hours. For example, if you wake up at 7 a.m., you could eat breakfast at 8 a.m., have lunch at noon, half a meal at 4 p.m., another half at 6 p.m., and a complete dinner (or half a dinner, depending on your hunger level) at 8 p.m. If you're still awake by midnight, you could eat a complete or half meal before bed. These choices are yours—there is no right or wrong way to do this, as long as you are tuned into your body.

- You can eat any meal at any time, i.e., breakfast for lunch. Make it your own and keep it simple for your lifestyle.

- Choose a lean protein and a fresh organic fruit or vegetable as your carbohydrate for each meal. You can cook vegetables; however, fresh and raw fruits and vegetables will yield the quickest weight loss on this program. If you buy conventionally grown produce, soak and wash the produce with a "veggie wash" to remove harmful chemicals, waxes, and soil. Or use a bath of kosher salt, a little vinegar, and warm water.

- Nutrition facts for each meal are listed within the meal plans. To personalize your portions, use your palm as a guide for your protein portion and your fist for your carbohydrate portion. You can cut your portions in half to substitute two snacks for a meal at any time.

- Choose a healthy fat such as extra virgin olive oil to cook with or to add flavor to your meal. Fat portions are approximately the size of a shot glass for nuts and half a shot glass for oils.

- Drink at least 10 glasses of water each day. Add a squirt of fresh lemon for added flavor and internal cleansing.

- Each day, drink at least 2 cups of cleansing tea, such as the Skinny Chicks' Detox Tea. To make, in a large saucepan, bring 5 cups water and 3 ounces fresh ginger, peeled and chopped, to a gentle boil. Remove from heat, add 6 bags dandelion root tea and 2 cinnamon sticks, cover, and steep for 15 minutes. Strain into a large pitcher, add 30 drops (one dose) artichoke extract and 2 tablespoons fresh lemon juice, stir, and chill in refrigerator. Enjoy throughout the day.

- Consume no more than 120 milligrams of caffeine (the equivalent of 1 cup of coffee or 3 cups of green tea) per day.

- Avoid alcoholic beverages, desserts, preservatives, and dining out as much as possible.

- Consume a minimum of three or four servings of fresh or frozen organically grown fruits and vegetables per day. See above for pointers on washing fruits and veggies.

- If you have access to a sauna and if you are not pregnant, sit in the sauna for 10 minutes each day. Toxins leave the body more readily when your core body temperature is elevated. This also promotes the release of human growth hormone, which is known to enhance youthfulness and foster better skin.

- Begin taking supplements: omega-3 fatty acids, a B-complex, and a multivitamin. These will help speed up your detox, especially the B-complex. (Try Simply Slimmer, my cutting-edge line of healthy supplements, available at www.christineavanti.com.)

- Repeat this plan for 1 to 4 weeks. Remember, you are free to mix and match all meals or repeat meals if need be. You can also mix and match the proteins, carbs, and fats among the meals.

As you will see, I have separated the nutrients out for you. That way you can learn which foods are rich in protein, carbs, and fat. The idea is to understand the predominant nutrient of each food you eat. Once you learn this, it becomes easy. Read through this meal plan carefully—learning the nutrients you get from foods is a cornerstone of your success.

There's also a box for "free foods"—foods so low in calories and sugar that it is unnecessary to count their calories. "Free foods" will not affect blood sugar levels, so enjoy! You can also find lists of my favorite proteins, carbs, fats, and free foods in the Appendix, starting on page 286.

Variety is the spice of life, and in nutrition, variety is also healthy. But if you only find two or three meals that work for you, for the sake of simplicity, feel free to eat mostly those during your weight loss period (and be sure to take the supplements I recommend in Chapter 12).

DAY 1

BREAKFAST

Pomegranate Blueberry Greek Yogurt

Combine all ingredients into a medium bowl and enjoy with a cup of Skinny Chicks' Detox Tea (see page 120).

Nutrition facts: 320 calories, 27 grams protein, 45 grams carbohydrates, 9 grams fat

PROTEIN POWERED	One 8-oz container 0% plain Greek yogurt
CARBOHYDRATE CONCENTRATED	¼ c pomegranate seeds, ¼ c blueberries, 1 Tbsp agave nectar
FAT FRIENDLY	1 Tbsp crushed walnuts
FREE FOODS	Water, tea, coffee

CHRISTINE'S NUTRITION NUGGETS Pomegranates and blueberries are loaded with antioxidants that help reduce the risk of cancer and heart disease. They also enhance the production of glutathione, one of the most potent antioxidants in the body. Glutathione improves liver function and detoxification.

LUNCH

Grilled Salmon or Turkey Burger on a Bed of Arugula with Lemon

Serve the grilled salmon or turkey burger on a bed of arugula drizzled with extra virgin olive oil mixed with lemon juice, a dab of Dijon, and minced garlic, with a side of wild rice and a peach.

Nutrition facts: 363 calories, 28 grams protein, 48 grams carbohydrates, 8 grams fat

PROTEIN POWERED	3-oz (uncooked) salmon or turkey patty
CARBOHYDRATE CONCENTRATED	¾ c cooked wild rice 1 peach
FAT FRIENDLY	1 tsp extra virgin olive oil, omega-3s in the salmon
FREE FOODS	1 c arugula Dab of Dijon mustard, lemon juice, and ¼ tsp minced garlic Water, tea

MIDAFTERNOON
High-Fiber, Low-Fat Protein Bar and Fruit
Grab and go!

Nutrition facts: 330 calories, 21 grams protein, 45 grams carbohydrates, 8 grams fat

PROTEIN POWERED	1 high-fiber, low-fat protein bar (such as Chocolate Clif Builder Bar)
CARBOHYDRATE CONCENTRATED	1 nectarine
FAT FRIENDLY	None; the fat in this meal comes in the protein bar.
FREE FOODS	Water, tea

DINNER
Oven-Roasted Chicken Breast, Rice or Quinoa, Carrots, and Zucchini
Pair oven-roasted chicken breast (prepared at home or store-bought) with brown rice or quinoa, steamed zucchini, and carrots. Munch on frozen grapes for a sweet ending.

Nutrition facts: 381 calories, 27 grams protein, 55 grams carbohydrates, 7 grams fat

PROTEIN POWERED	3 oz oven-roasted skinless chicken breast
CARBOHYDRATE CONCENTRATED	³/₄ c cooked brown rice or quinoa ½ c steamed carrots ½ c frozen grapes
FAT FRIENDLY	1 tsp extra virgin olive oil
FREE FOODS	Your choice of herbs and spices 1 c steamed zucchini Water, tea

DAY 2

BREAKFAST

Huevos Rancheros (with Potatoes Instead of Tortillas) (At Home or Dining Out)

To make at home, see the recipe on page 245.

Nutrition facts: 343 calories, 25 grams protein, 44 grams carbohydrates, 7 grams fat

PROTEIN POWERED	Egg whites (fresh or use Eggology brand) Nonfat cheese
CARBOHYDRATE CONCENTRATED	Potatoes Enchilada sauce
FAT FRIENDLY	Extra virgin olive oil
FREE FOODS	Onions, cilantro Water, tea, coffee

LUNCH

Baked Yam Stuffed with Peanut Butter, Cottage Cheese, and Cinnamon

Wash and dry yam, then wrap with plastic and microwave 5–6 min. Remove plastic and slice yam lengthwise. Spread with peanut butter. Add cottage cheese, sprinkled with cinnamon and a drizzle of agave nectar.

Nutrition facts: 358 calories, 23 grams protein, 46 grams carbohydrates, 11 grams fat

PROTEIN POWERED	³/₄ c low-fat, low-sodium cottage cheese
CARBOHYDRATE CONCENTRATED	Small yam (approx 4–5 oz) 1 tsp agave nectar
FAT FRIENDLY	1 Tbsp natural peanut butter
FREE FOODS	Cinnamon Water, tea

MIDAFTERNOON
Hard-Boiled Eggs, Yogurt, and Fruit

Mix sliced bananas with yogurt. Enjoy with eggs on the side.

Nutrition facts: 355 calories, 20 grams protein, 48 grams carbohydrates, 10 grams fat

PROTEIN POWERED	2 hard-boiled omega-3 eggs
CARBOHYDRATE CONCENTRATED	One 6-oz container nonfat flavored yogurt 1 small banana, sliced
FAT FRIENDLY	There are 10 grams of fat in the eggs. Thus, no additional fat is needed.
FREE FOODS	Water, tea

DINNER
Coconut Curry Sea Bass over Red Lentils

See recipe on page 266.

Nutrition facts: 344 calories, 25 grams protein, 42 grams carbohydrates, 9 grams fat

PROTEIN POWERED	Sea bass
CARBOHYDRATE CONCENTRATED	Red lentils
FAT FRIENDLY	Extra virgin olive oil cooking spray Light coconut milk Coconut flakes
FREE FOODS	Red onion Cilantro Minced garlic Yellow curry powder Water, tea

CHRISTINE'S NUTRITION NUGGETS According to a 2007 study from Purdue University, increased protein intake improved satiety at meals. What's more, protein provides important amino acids needed by the liver for detoxification, such as methionine and cysteine.

DAY 3

BREAKFAST
Wild Berry Parfait

Mix cottage cheese, strawberries, blueberries, and berry yogurt; sprinkle with flaxseed or walnuts. Serve with a cup of Skinny Chicks' Detox Tea (see page 120), plain or sweetened with a small drop of agave nectar.

Nutrition facts: 317 calories, 22 grams protein, 45 grams carbohydrates, 7 grams fat

PROTEIN POWERED	³/₄ c low-fat, low-sodium cottage cheese
CARBOHYDRATE CONCENTRATED	¹/₂ c each of strawberries and blueberries One 6-oz container berry-flavored light yogurt
FAT FRIENDLY	2 Tbsp ground flaxseed or 1 Tbsp crushed walnuts
FREE FOODS	Water, tea, coffee

LUNCH
Egg White Salad in Lettuce Cups and Fruit Salad

In a medium bowl, combine eggs, mayo, green onion, celery, vinegar, and salt and pepper to taste. Spoon egg salad into lettuce cups. Serve with mixed organic fruits.

Nutrition facts: 333 calories, 20 grams protein, 44 grams carbohydrates, 11 grams fat

PROTEIN POWERED	5 hard-boiled egg whites, chopped
CARBOHYDRATE CONCENTRATED	¹/₂ c sliced fresh mango ¹/₂ c pineapple
FAT FRIENDLY	2 Tbsp light mayo
FREE FOODS	1 Tbsp minced green onion 1 Tbsp diced celery 1 tsp cider vinegar Salt and ground black pepper Water, tea

MIDAFTERNOON
Citrus-y Greek Yogurt

Mix yogurt, sliced orange sections, and walnuts in a medium bowl. Garnish with fresh mint leaf.

Nutrition facts: 332 calories, 28 grams protein, 47 grams carbohydrates, 5 grams fat

PROTEIN POWERED	One 8-oz container 0% plain Greek yogurt
CARBOHYDRATE CONCENTRATED	1 large orange 1 Tbsp agave nectar
FAT FRIENDLY	2 Tbsp ground flaxseed or 1 Tbsp crushed nuts
FREE FOODS	Mint leaf Water, tea

DINNER
Herb-Crusted Salmon with Baby Potatoes and Artichokes

Steam artichoke over low heat for 30–40 minutes. Preheat oven to 350°F. Line a baking tray with foil and spray with olive oil. Wash salmon, pat dry, and spread garlic, rosemary, salt, and pepper over top. Bake for 10–15 min, depending on thickness. Serve with artichoke, steamed spinach, and boiled potatoes.

Nutrition facts: 371 calories, 28 grams protein, 52 grams carbohydrates, 8 grams fat

PROTEIN POWERED	3 oz salmon
CARBOHYDRATE CONCENTRATED	6 oz red potatoes 1 medium steamed artichoke
FAT FRIENDLY	Extra virgin olive oil cooking spray
FREE FOODS	1 c spinach 1 Tbsp minced garlic 1 Tbsp minced rosemary Salt and ground black pepper Water, tea

CHRISTINE'S NUTRITION NUGGETS Artichokes have active compounds called caffeoylquinic acids or cynarin that prevent the buildup of fat and toxins in the liver. These compounds also act as a gentle laxative by increasing bile secretion.

DAY 4

BREAKFAST

Spinach and Feta Scramble (At Home or Dining Out)

To make at home, sauté spinach in a pan coated with olive oil cooking spray, add egg whites, and scramble until cooked. Add feta, basil, and tomato. For potatoes, wash, slice, sprinkle with salt and pepper to taste. Place in a glass bowl and cover with plastic wrap. Microwave 2 ½ min. Enjoy a cup of Skinny Chicks' Detox Tea (see page 120) plain or sweetened with a small drop of agave nectar and a small shot glass of pomegranate juice. If ordering out, omit the cheese.

Nutrition facts: 319 calories, 23 grams protein, 46 grams carbohydrates, 5 grams fat

PROTEIN POWERED	4 egg whites 2 Tbsp fat-free feta
CARBOHYDRATE CONCENTRATED	¼ c pomegranate juice 2 small baby red potatoes
FAT FRIENDLY	Extra virgin olive oil cooking spray
FREE FOODS	½ c spinach leaves 1 basil leaf Tomato, diced Salt and ground black pepper Water, tea, coffee

LUNCH

Tuna-Stuffed Celery Sticks with Fruit

In a medium bowl, combine tuna, egg, black olives, mayo, mustard, vinegar, and onion. Season with salt and pepper to taste. Stuff tuna salad into celery sticks and enjoy with a fresh peach and pomegranate juice.

Nutrition facts: 340 calories, 22 grams protein, 42 grams carbohydrates, 10 grams fat

PROTEIN POWERED	2 oz chunky light tuna 1 hard-boiled egg, diced
CARBOHYDRATE CONCENTRATED	Peach ½ c pomegranate juice
FAT FRIENDLY	1 Tbsp diced black olives 1 Tbsp light mayo
FREE FOODS	4 stalks celery 1 tsp diced onion 1 tsp red wine vinegar 1 tsp Dijon mustard Salt and ground black pepper Water, tea

MIDAFTERNOON
Pumpkin Pie Cottage Cheese

Combine all ingredients in a medium bowl. Mix well. Sprinkle with cinnamon and enjoy.

Nutrition facts: 333 calories, 23 grams protein, 49 grams carbohydrates, 8 grams fat

PROTEIN POWERED	$^3/_4$ c low-fat, low-sodium cottage cheese
CARBOHYDRATE CONCENTRATED	$^1/_2$ c canned organic pumpkin puree 2 Tbsp raisins 2 Tbsp agave nectar
FAT FRIENDLY	2 Tbsp ground flaxseed
FREE FOODS	Cinnamon Water, tea

CHRISTINE'S NUTRITION NUGGETS The insoluble fiber in ground flaxseed acts as a natural laxative and increases regularity and elimination of toxins.

DINNER
Grilled White Fish with Quinoa or Brown Rice and Asparagus

Preheat grill to medium. Spray fish with olive oil spray, then rub with herbs and spices. Spray asparagus with olive oil spray and sprinkle with herbs and spices. Grill fish and asparagus until fish flakes easily with a fork. Serve with quinoa or brown rice. Finish with agave nectar–sweetened raspberries.

Nutrition facts: 360 calories, 28 grams protein, 47 grams carbohydrates, 9 grams fat

PROTEIN POWERED	$3^1/_2$ oz of white fish (any variety)
CARBOHYDRATE CONCENTRATED	$^1/_2$ c cooked quinoa or brown rice $^3/_4$ c raspberries 2 tsp agave nectar
FAT FRIENDLY	Extra virgin olive oil cooking spray
FREE FOODS	Your favorite herbs and spices Asparagus spears (add salt and pepper to taste) Water, tea

DAY 5

BREAKFAST

Blueberry Peach Smoothie

Combine blueberries, peaches, protein powder, ice cubes, water, and almond butter in a blender. Blend until thick and smooth. Enjoy with a cup of Skinny Chicks' Detox Tea (see page 120), plain or sweetened with a small drop of agave nectar.

Nutrition facts: 377 calories, 26 grams protein, 54 grams carbohydrates, 10 grams fat

PROTEIN POWERED	1 scoop vanilla-flavored protein powder
CARBOHYDRATE CONCENTRATED	1¼ c frozen blueberries 1½ c frozen peaches
FAT FRIENDLY	1 Tbsp natural almond butter or 2 tsp flaxseed oil
FREE FOODS	8 ice cubes 1–2 c water Tea, coffee

CHRISTINE'S NUTRITION NUGGETS All fruit is naturally low in fat, sodium, and calories. Blueberries contain phytochemicals called anthocyanidins and proanthocyanins, which may play a role in preserving memory.

LUNCH

BBQ Chicken Breast, Corn Cobbette, and Melon

BBQ the chicken however you like, prepare corn in boiling water or on grill, add salt to taste. Enjoy with a side of cantaloupe.

Nutrition facts: 393 calories, 27 grams protein, 50 grams carbohydrates, 12 grams fat

PROTEIN POWERED	3 oz BBQ skinless chicken breast
CARBOHYDRATE CONCENTRATED	½ ear of corn 2 cantaloupe wedges (or 2 c cubed melon)
FAT FRIENDLY	1 tsp extra virgin olive oil (brush onto chicken before grilling)
FREE FOODS	1 Tbsp BBQ sauce Water, tea

MIDAFTERNOON
Turkey and Cheese Roll-Up

Wrap deli slices around cheese sticks and dip into Dijon mustard. Enjoy with grapefruit and sweet cherries.

Nutrition facts: 359 calories, 24 grams protein, 58 grams carbohydrates, 10 grams fat

PROTEIN POWERED	2 sticks reduced-fat string cheese 2 slices low-sodium deli turkey
CARBOHYDRATE CONCENTRATED	1 large grapefruit ³/₄ c fresh cherries
FAT FRIENDLY	No need to add fat because there is fat in the string cheese.
FREE FOODS	Dijon mustard Water, tea

DINNER
Cilantro Lime Sea Bass

See recipe on page 267, exchanging the couscous for brown rice.

Nutrition facts per serving: 350 calories, 22 grams protein, 49 grams carbohydrates, 10 grams fat

PROTEIN POWERED	Sea bass
CARBOHYDRATE CONCENTRATED	Brown rice
FAT FRIENDLY	Extra virgin olive oil
FREE FOODS	Lime juice, cilantro, ginger Water, tea

DAY 6

BREAKFAST

Veggie Delight Scramble

Wash potatoes and wrap in plastic wrap. Microwave 4 min. Heat stove to medium. In a medium skillet coated with olive oil cooking spray, sauté onions, mushrooms, and spinach 2 min. Add egg whites and scramble until mostly cooked. Add diced tomato and cheddar and season with salt and pepper to taste. Serve with potatoes. Enjoy with a cup of Skinny Chicks' Detox Tea (see page 120), plain or sweetened with a small drop of agave nectar.

Nutrition facts: 327 calories, 25 grams protein, 46 grams carbohydrates, 5 grams fat

PROTEIN POWERED	4 egg whites 2 Tbsp fat-free Cheddar
CARBOHYDRATE CONCENTRATED	2 baby potatoes 1½ c cubed watermelon
FAT FRIENDLY	Extra virgin olive oil cooking spray
FREE FOODS	1 Tbsp diced onions ¼ c sliced mushrooms ¼ c spinach 1 Tbsp diced tomato Salt and ground black pepper Water, tea, coffee

DINING OUT LUNCH

Sushi, Brown Rice, and Steamed Veggies

Order at your favorite sushi hot spot!

Nutrition facts: 326 calories, 22 grams protein, 44 grams carbohydrates, 4 grams fat

PROTEIN POWERED	2 pieces salmon roll 2 pieces tuna roll* 2 pieces yellowtail roll *If pregnant, swap tuna for salmon.
CARBOHYDRATE CONCENTRATED	Sushi is wrapped in rice, thus no need to add any other carbs to this meal.
FAT FRIENDLY	⅕ avocado, diced (rolled into sushi)
FREE FOODS	Low-sodium soy sauce, wasabi 1 c steamed veggies Water, tea

MIDAFTERNOON
Low-Sodium Deli Slices and Fruit

Combine mayo with honey mustard for dipping deli slices. Enjoy with 2 pieces of fresh summer fruit.

Nutrition facts: 318 calories, 17 grams protein, 44 grams carbohydrates, 8 grams fat

PROTEIN POWERED	3 low-sodium deli slices (turkey, ham, or chicken)
CARBOHYDRATE CONCENTRATED	1 large peach 1 large nectarine
FAT FRIENDLY	1 Tbsp light mayo
FREE FOODS	1 Tbsp honey mustard Water, tea

DINNER
Cajun-Style Grilled Shrimp and Brown Rice

See recipe on page 268.

Nutrition facts per serving: 410 calories, 28 grams protein, 50 grams carbohydrates, 11 grams fat

PROTEIN POWERED	Grilled shrimp
CARBOHYDRATE CONCENTRATED	Brown rice
FAT FRIENDLY	Extra virgin olive oil
FREE FOODS	Lemon juice Herbs and spices Water, tea

CHRISTINE'S NUTRITION NUGGETS Sushi is a healthy and delicious food; however, there are concerns of mercury in large predator fish such as bigeye and ahi tuna used for sushi. According to government data, these fish contain medium mercury levels (approximately 0.6 microgram per gram). The FDA says it's safe for women of childbearing age to consume two servings of tuna per week; however, I recommend avoiding tuna until you are through breastfeeding.

DAY 7

BREAKFAST

Steel-Cut Oats with a Side of Sweet Yogurt

Prepare oats in water, according to package directions. Top with fresh strawberry slices. Enjoy with a side of Greek yogurt drizzled with agave nectar and a cup of Skinny Chicks' Detox Tea (see page 120), plain or sweetened with a small drop of agave nectar.

Nutrition facts: 347 calories, 25 grams protein, 49 grams carbohydrates, 6 grams fat

PROTEIN POWERED	6 oz 0% plain Greek yogurt
CARBOHYDRATE CONCENTRATED	1 c cooked steel-cut oats (1/2 c dry) 2 tsp agave nectar 1/4 c sliced strawberries
FAT FRIENDLY	2 Tbsp ground flaxseed or 1 Tbsp slivered almonds
FREE FOODS	Water, tea, coffee

LUNCH

Baked Turkey Breast, Sweet Potato, and Zucchini (At Home or Dining Out)

To make at home, roast turkey breast or reheat store-bought. Wrap sweet potato in plastic wrap and microwave 6–7 min. Remove plastic wrap and slice lengthwise. Sprinkle with brown sugar. Steam zucchini with garlic salt and pepper.

Nutrition facts: 398 calories, 32 grams protein, 56 grams carbohydrates, 6 grams fat

PROTEIN POWERED	3 oz roasted skinless turkey breast
CARBOHYDRATE CONCENTRATED	1 medium (6-oz) sweet potato 1 tsp brown sugar
FAT FRIENDLY	Extra virgin olive oil cooking spray
FREE FOODS	Zucchini Garlic salt and ground black pepper Water, tea

MIDAFTERNOON
California Fruit Kebabs

See recipe on page 280. Sprinkle with nuts

Nutrition facts per serving: 313 calories, 27 grams protein, 46 grams carbohydrates, 4 grams fat

PROTEIN POWERED	One 8-oz container 0% plain Greek yogurt
CARBOHYDRATE CONCENTRATED	Watermelon, honeydew melon, cantaloupe, strawberries, honey
FAT FRIENDLY	1 Tbsp slivered almonds Cooking spray
FREE FOODS	Mint, water, tea

DINNER
Tex-Mex Chicken with Chipotle Sauce

See recipe on page 275.

Nutrition facts per serving: 380 calories, 24 grams protein, 49 grams carbohydrates, 11 grams fat

PROTEIN POWERED	3 oz chicken breast
CARBOHYDRATE CONCENTRATED	Black beans, corn
FAT FRIENDLY	Avocado, olive oil Cooking spray
FREE FOODS	Cilantro, lime, pepper, onion, tomatoes, jalapeño Water, tea

CHRISTINE'S NUTRITION NUGGETS Oats are a fantastic source of soluble fiber (which absorbs water; insoluble fiber does not). Soluble fiber helps to stabilize blood sugar levels, lowers cholesterol, and curbs hunger. Soluble fiber also soaks up toxins in the intestines and moves them out of the body. Soluble fiber can also be found in apples, pears, grapefruits, and artichokes.

The Skinny Chicks Everyday Weight Loss Plan

My general weight loss program differs from the kick-start in that you will be allowed to enjoy whole grain breads, crackers, cereal, and pasta. Each meal is designed as a fat-burning PC Combo. Don't feel confused by all the options. Again, variety is healthy, but if you find two or three meals you love, feel free to eat those as often as you like during your weight loss period (and be sure to take the supplements I recommend in Chapter 12). If you have a large amount of body fat to lose and you hit a plateau at any point on the Skinny Chicks everyday program, you may have too many toxins in your bloodstream. Returning to the kick-start plan for a week will help get your fat burning going again.

Most of the meals on this plan can be ordered at a restaurant; just remember to ask your server to omit any cheeses, creams or cream sauces, guacamole, gravies, or mayo. If they forget, you should remove or scrape off these items yourself. I have also included simple grab-and-go meals.

Everyday Meal Plan Guidelines

- Choose a lean protein, a healthy carbohydrate, and fat for each meal.
- Eat a PC Combo every 4 hours, keeping the total calories for each below 400.
- Can't eat every 4 hours? Simply cut the meal portions in half and eat every 2 hours. For example, if you wake up at 7 a.m., you could eat breakfast at 8 a.m., have lunch at noon, half a meal at 4 p.m., another half at 6 p.m., and a complete dinner (or half a dinner, depending on your hunger level) at 8 p.m. If you're still awake by midnight, you could eat a complete or half meal before bed. These choices are yours—there is no right or wrong way to do this, as long as you are tuned into your body.
- Mix and match meals as you like. You can have breakfast for lunch and dinner for breakfast—whatever works best for your lifestyle.
- Remember to use your palm as a guide for your protein portion and your fist for your carbohydrate portion. (Or you can use the measurements listed.)

- Recall that you are free to cut your portions in half to substitute two snacks for a meal at any time.

- Choose a healthy fat to cook with or to add flavor to your meal. Fat portions are approximately the size of a shot glass for nuts and half a shot glass for oils.

- Drink at least 10 glasses of water each day.

- Consume no more than 120 milligrams of caffeine (the equivalent of 1 cup of coffee or 3 cups of green tea) each day.

- Avoid alcoholic beverages, desserts, preservatives, and dining out as much as possible.

- If you choose to have an alcoholic beverage or dessert, be sure to reduce your meal portions.

- Consume a minimum of three to four servings of fresh or frozen organically grown fruits and vegetables per day. If you buy conventionally grown produce, soak and wash it with a "veggie wash" to remove harmful chemicals. If you don't have veggie wash, you can use a solution of kosher salt, vinegar, and warm water. (Make this a habit in general, not only while you are on this program!)

- Be sure to take supplements: omega-3 fatty acids, B-complex, and a multivitamin. All of these are available at my Web site, www.christineavanti.com. These will help speed up your detox, especially the B-complex.

- Once weight loss goals are reached, continue to eat PC Combos to maintain weight loss results and overall good health, allowing yourself up to 450 calories per meal if you like.

As you will see, I have separated the nutrients out for you so you can learn the predominant nutrients of your foods. Once you learn this, it becomes easy. Remember that you can mix and match different kinds of proteins, carbs, and fats if you like.

The "free foods"—foods that are so low in calories and sugar that it is unnecessary to count their calories—will not affect blood sugar levels, so enjoy. You can also find lists of my favorite proteins, carbs, fats, and free foods in the Appendix.

DAY 1

BREAKFAST

Apple Maple Pecan Parfait

Combine all ingredients in a medium bowl and enjoy.

Nutrition facts: 384 calories, 26 grams protein, 56 grams carbohydrates, 8 grams fat

PROTEIN POWERED	¾ c low-fat, low-sodium cottage cheese
CARBOHYDRATE CONCENTRATED	1 6-oz container light vanilla yogurt 1 Tbsp maple syrup ½ medium apple, diced
FAT FRIENDLY	2 Tbsp crushed pecans
FREE FOODS	Water, tea, coffee

LUNCH

Turkey Sandwich, Baby Carrots, and Fruit

Place turkey between bread slices, spread with avocado and Dijon mustard, and add your favorite "free" veggies. Munch on baby carrots and apricots on the side. Enjoy!

Nutrition facts: 395 calories, 25 grams protein, 51 grams carbohydrates, 11 grams fat

PROTEIN POWERED	3 slices low-sodium smoked deli turkey
CARBOHYDRATE CONCENTRATED	2 slices whole grain bread, toasted 2 small apricots 10 baby carrots
FAT FRIENDLY	⅕ medium Hass avocado
FREE FOODS	Dijon mustard Baby spinach leaves Tomato Red onion Water, tea

MIDAFTERNOON
Grilled Chicken Cilantro Lime Wrap

Pile chicken and vegetables on a tortilla and top with fresh lime juice, cilantro, and salsa. Wrap and roll and enjoy with mango on the side.

Nutrition facts: 373 calories, 26 grams protein, 47 grams carbohydrates, 10 grams fat

PROTEIN POWERED	3 oz grilled skinless chicken breast
CARBOHYDRATE CONCENTRATED	1 medium whole wheat tortilla or pita $1/2$ c fresh mango slices
FAT FRIENDLY	Olive oil cooking spray $1/5$ medium Hass avocado
FREE FOODS	Lime juice Chopped cilantro Diced tomato Shredded lettuce Salsa Water, tea

DINNER
Filet Mignon with Mushroom Sauce and Herbed Mashed Potatoes

See recipe on page 278, substituting filet mignon for the sirloin.

Nutrition facts per serving: 361 calories, 24 grams protein, 50 grams carbohydrates, 6 grams fat

PROTEIN POWERED	Filet mignon
CARBOHYDRATE CONCENTRATED	Potatoes
FAT FRIENDLY	Extra virgin olive oil
FREE FOODS	Mushrooms Garlic, rosemary, thyme Chicken broth Water, tea

CHRISTINE'S NUTRITION NUGGETS Feel free to munch on "free foods"—such as cucumber slices seasoned with rice vinegar, salt, and freshly ground black pepper—between meals if you feel hungry. A nice warm cup of fruit-flavored tea will also be enjoyable between meals. Tea contains an amino acid called L-theanine that has been proven to increase the activity of alpha brain waves, which increases awareness and calmness.

DAY 2

BREAKFAST

Protein-Powered Vanilla French Toast

See recipe on page 244.

Nutrition facts per serving: 360 calories, 25 grams protein, 47 grams carbohydrates, 7 grams fat

PROTEIN POWERED	Protein powder Egg whites
CARBOHYDRATE CONCENTRATED	Whole wheat bread
FAT FRIENDLY	Omega-3 spread
FREE FOODS	Vanilla extract Fat-free whipped topping Water, tea, coffee

LUNCH

Chicken Soft Taco (At Home or Dining Out)

Wrap chicken into warm tortilla with lettuce, tomato, onion, and salsa. Enjoy black beans and rice on the side. If dining out, order two chicken soft tacos and request no cheese, no sour cream, and no special sauces except for salsa.

Nutrition facts: 388 calories, 29 grams protein, 56 grams carbohydrates, 7 grams fat

PROTEIN POWERED	3 oz grilled skinless chicken breast
CARBOHYDRATE CONCENTRATED	One 6" whole wheat tortilla 1/4 c black beans 1/4 c rice
FAT FRIENDLY	Extra virgin olive oil cooking spray
FREE FOODS	Shredded lettuce Tomato Onion Fresh salsa Water, tea

MIDAFTERNOON
Apple Cinnamon Cottage Cheese

Combine all ingredients in a medium bowl, and mix well. Enjoy!

Nutrition facts: 338 calories, 22 grams protein, 47 grams carbohydrates, 7 grams fat

PROTEIN POWERED	¾ c low-fat, low-sodium cottage cheese
CARBOHYDRATE CONCENTRATED	¾ c unsweetened organic applesauce
FAT FRIENDLY	1 pinch slivered almonds
FREE FOODS	Cinnamon Water, tea

DINNER
Christine's Pasta and Spicy Red Sauce

See recipe on page 259.

Nutrition facts per serving: 425 calories, 31 grams protein, 59 grams carbohydrates, 9 grams fat

PROTEIN POWERED	4 oz extra-lean ground turkey Reduced-fat Parmesan cheese
CARBOHYDRATE CONCENTRATED	1 c cooked whole wheat pasta Tomato sauce
FAT FRIENDLY	Extra virgin olive oil
FREE FOODS	Onion Bell pepper Garlic Diced tomatoes Water, tea

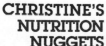

CHRISTINE'S NUTRITION NUGGETS Tomatoes are loaded with lycopene, a powerful antioxidant that has been proven to reduce the risk of cardiovascular disease and prostate and gastrointestinal cancers. So load up on that red sauce!

DAY 3

BREAKFAST

Southwest Scramble with Corn Tortillas (At Home or Dining Out)

To make at home, see recipe on page 248.

Nutrition facts per serving: 382 calories, 25 grams protein, 50 grams carbohydrates, 9 grams fat

PROTEIN POWERED	Egg whites Low-fat Mexican cheese
CARBOHYDRATE CONCENTRATED	Corn tortillas Fresh corn
FAT FRIENDLY	Omega-3 spread
FREE FOODS	Green chile peppers Scallions Salsa (optional) Water, tea, coffee

LUNCH

Cheese and Veggie Quesadilla

Coat a medium frying pan with cooking spray. Warm tortilla over medium heat until it begins to brown. Add shredded cheese. Once cheese is melted, add your favorite free veggies and condiments and serve.

Nutrition facts: 346 calories, 24 grams protein, 52 grams carbohydrates, 5 grams fat

PROTEIN POWERED	$1/2$ c fat-free shredded Cheddar or mozzarella cheese
CARBOHYDRATE CONCENTRATED	One 6" whole wheat or corn tortilla 1 large watermelon wedge (or 1 c cubed)
FAT FRIENDLY	$1/5$ medium Hass avocado Extra virgin olive oil cooking spray
FREE FOODS	Tomato Onion Salsa 1 Tbsp fat-free sour cream Water, tea

MIDAFTERNOON
Turkey Jerky, Cherries, and Trail Mix

Grab and go!

Nutrition facts: 334 calories, 20 grams protein, 42 grams carbohydrates, 13 grams fat

PROTEIN POWERED	1 oz turkey jerky (I like Snack Masters brand)
CARBOHYDRATE CONCENTRATED	1 c fresh cherries ¼ c unsalted trail mix
FAT FRIENDLY	Nuts in the trail mix
FREE FOODS	Water, tea

DINNER
Wasabi Sesame Salmon with Brown Rice Noodles

See recipe on page 263.

Nutrition facts per serving: 400 calories, 25 grams protein, 48 grams carbohydrates, 12 grams fat

PROTEIN POWERED	Salmon
CARBOHYDRATE CONCENTRATED	Brown rice spaghetti Carrots
FAT FRIENDLY	Light mayo Sesame seeds
FREE FOODS	Wasabi, soy sauce, chicken broth, chili sauce Scallions

CHRISTINE'S NUTRITION NUGGETS Salmon is packed with heart-healthy omega-3 fatty acids, which are known to lower blood pressure.

DAY 4
BREAKFAST
Peanut Butter Toast

Spread peanut butter on toast and place ¼ c cottage cheese on each slice of toast. Sprinkle with cinnamon and enjoy with ½ banana on the side.

Nutrition facts: 359 calories, 23 grams protein, 43 grams carbohydrates, 11 grams fat

PROTEIN POWERED	½ c low-fat, low-sodium cottage cheese
CARBOHYDRATE CONCENTRATED	2 slices whole grain bread or 1 whole wheat English muffin ½ small banana
FAT FRIENDLY	1 Tbsp natural peanut butter
FREE FOODS	Cinnamon Water, tea, coffee

LUNCH
Blue Ribbon Cheeseburger (At Home or Dining Out)

Spread toasted bun with Dijon mustard and light mayo, then add turkey patty, blue cheese, lettuce, tomato, and onion. Garnish with a pickle. Enjoy with a fresh wedge of watermelon. If dining out, omit the cheese; if fresh fruit is not available, replace with a small lemonade.

Nutrition facts: 412 calories, 30 grams protein, 57 grams carbohydrates, 9 grams fat

PROTEIN POWERED	1 low-fat turkey burger patty 1 Tbsp reduced-fat blue cheese
CARBOHYDRATE CONCENTRATED	1 whole wheat bun 1 large watermelon wedge, or 1 c cubed
FAT FRIENDLY	Extra virgin olive oil cooking spray (for grilling) 1 Tbsp light mayo
FREE FOODS	Dijon mustard Lettuce Tomato Onion Pickle Water, tea

MIDAFTERNOON
Citrus-y Greek Yogurt

See recipe on page 127. Cut orange into segments and combine in a medium bowl with remaining ingredients. Garnish with fresh mint leaf and enjoy.

Nutrition facts: 332 calories, 28 grams protein, 47 grams carbohydrates, 5 grams fat

CHRISTINE'S NUTRITION NUGGETS Low-fat dairy products contain higher amounts of protein, vitamin D, and calcium, and less disease-causing saturated fat.

DINNER
Grilled Chicken Fajitas

See recipe on page 274 or order at your favorite Tex-Mex restaurant. A portion should be two 6" tortillas filled with ingredients.

Nutrition facts per serving: 417 calories, 30 grams protein, 56 grams carbohydrates, 8 grams fat

PROTEIN POWERED	Grilled skinless chicken breast
CARBOHYDRATE CONCENTRATED	Whole wheat or corn tortillas
FAT FRIENDLY	Extra virgin olive oil cooking spray
FREE FOODS	Bell pepper Onion Tomato Salsa Lime juice Fat-free sour cream Water, tea

DAY 5

BREAKFAST
Berry Delish Oatmeal

Prepare oats in water according to package directions. Add protein powder immediately after cooking. Top with berries, agave nectar, and slivered almonds, and sprinkle with cinnamon.

Nutrition facts: 366 calories, 23 grams protein, 56 grams carbohydrates, 7 grams fat

PROTEIN POWERED	½ scoop protein powder ½ c nonfat milk or soy milk
CARBOHYDRATE CONCENTRATED	1 c cooked oats ¼ c blueberries, fresh or frozen ¼ c strawberries, fresh or frozen 2 tsp agave nectar
FAT FRIENDLY	1 Tbsp slivered almonds
FREE FOODS	Cinnamon Water, tea, coffee

LUNCH
Greek Chicken Pita with Cucumber and Mint

Spread hummus inside pita. Stuff chicken, cucumber, onion, tomato, and mint into pita. Season with vinegar, seasoning salt, and pepper and drizzle lightly with extra virgin olive oil. Enjoy with fresh grapes.

Nutrition facts: 401 calories, 28 grams protein, 54 grams carbohydrates, 10 grams fat

PROTEIN POWERED	2½ oz grilled skinless chicken breast 1 Tbsp fat-free feta cheese
CARBOHYDRATE CONCENTRATED	Whole wheat pita ½ c seedless grapes
FAT FRIENDLY	1 Tbsp hummus 1 tsp extra virgin olive oil
FREE FOODS	Cucumber, red onion, tomato Fresh mint leaves Red wine vinegar Seasoning salt and freshly cracked black pepper Water, tea

MIDAFTERNOON
Low-Fat Egg White Salad and Crackers

In a medium bowl, combine egg whites, mayo, bell pepper, onion, vinegar, and salt to taste. Serve with crackers and fresh strawberries.

Nutrition facts: 403 calories, 26 grams protein, 52 grams carbohydrates, 10 grams fat

PROTEIN POWERED	5 hard-boiled egg whites
CARBOHYDRATE CONCENTRATED	20 mini whole wheat crackers (I like Kashi TLC) 10 strawberries
FAT FRIENDLY	1 Tbsp light mayo
FREE FOODS	1 Tbsp minced green bell pepper 1 Tbsp minced red onion 1 tsp cider vinegar Salt Water, tea

DINNER
Mediterranean Shrimp Pasta

See recipe on page 261. Or order out: Ask for pasta with a broth-based sauce and grilled shrimp. Eat half of the restaurant portion.

Nutrition facts per serving: 399 calories, 30 grams protein, 48 grams carbohydrates, 10 grams fat

PROTEIN POWERED	Shrimp
CARBOHYDRATE CONCENTRATED	Brown rice pasta
FAT FRIENDLY	Extra virgin olive oil
FREE FOODS	Tomatoes Spinach Garlic Lemon Basil Water, tea

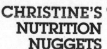 **CHRISTINE'S NUTRITION NUGGETS** Garlic is loaded with allyl sulfides, which have been proven to reduce the risk of cancer in multiple research studies.

DAY 6

BREAKFAST

Onion and Tomato Egg White Scramble
(At Home or Dining Out)

To make at home, heat range on medium low. Coat a medium pan with cooking spray. Add sliced green onion, salt, and pepper and sauté for 2 min. Add egg whites and scramble until almost cooked. Add diced tomato and fat-free cheese. Serve with 1 toasted waffle spread lightly with peanut butter.

Nutrition facts: 325 calories, 23 grams protein, 44 grams carbohydrates, 6 grams fat

PROTEIN POWERED	5 egg whites 1 oz fat-free cheese
CARBOHYDRATE CONCENTRATED	1 low-fat whole wheat frozen waffle 1 c orange juice
FAT FRIENDLY	Extra virgin olive oil cooking spray 1 Tbsp natural peanut butter
FREE FOODS	Green onion Tomato Salt and ground black pepper Water, tea, coffee

LUNCH

Veggie and Cheese Sandwich

Spread mashed avocado and light mayo on each slice of bread. Add your favorite "free" vegetables and enjoy with fresh apricots or any small fruit.

Nutrition facts: 371 calories, 26 grams protein, 47 grams carbohydrates, 8 grams fat

PROTEIN POWERED	3 slices or 2 oz fat-free cheese
CARBOHYDRATE CONCENTRATED	2 slices whole wheat bread 1 Tbsp shredded carrots 3 small apricots
FAT FRIENDLY	1 Tbsp mashed avocado 1 Tbsp light mayo
FREE FOODS	Cucumber, sprouts, spinach leaves, red onion, tomato Water, tea

MIDAFTERNOON

Grilled Salmon Burger with Arugula

Spread toasted bun with Dijon and top with grilled salmon patty, arugula, tomato, and onion. Garnish with cornichons. Enjoy with a delicious pomegranate.

Nutrition facts: 399 calories, 27 grams protein, 55 grams carbohydrates, 4 grams fat

PROTEIN POWERED	1 salmon patty
CARBOHYDRATE CONCENTRATED	1 whole wheat bun 1 fresh medium pomegranate
FAT FRIENDLY	The salmon burger contains healthy fat.
FREE FOODS	Dijon mustard Arugula, tomato, red onion Cornichons Water, tea

CHRISTINE'S NUTRITION NUGGETS Arugula is packed with vitamin A—about 10 percent of your recommended daily intake, or RDI, per cup. Vitamin A is beneficial in preventing night blindness, skin disorders, and even acne.

DINNER

Christine's Enchiladas

See recipe on page 277. Allow two enchiladas and ½ c rice per serving.

Nutrition facts per serving: 372 calories, 28 grams protein, 54 grams carbohydrates, 7 grams fat

PROTEIN POWERED	Extra-lean ground turkey Fat-free Cheddar cheese
CARBOHYDRATE CONCENTRATED	Tortillas Rice
FAT FRIENDLY	Extra virgin olive oil
FREE FOODS	Cilantro, onion, green chile peppers, garlic, red-pepper flakes, spices, salsa, fat-free sour cream Water, tea

DAY 7

BREAKFAST

Blueberry Yogurt Parfait with Slivered Almonds

In a medium bowl, combine all ingredients and mix well. Enjoy!

Nutrition facts: 308 calories, 22 grams protein, 46 grams carbohydrates, 5 grams fat

PROTEIN POWERED	½ c low-fat, low-sodium cottage cheese
CARBOHYDRATE CONCENTRATED	1 6-oz container light yogurt Handful or ½ c blueberries
FAT FRIENDLY	1 Tbsp slivered almonds
FREE FOODS	Water, tea, coffee

LUNCH

Grilled Chicken Sandwich (At Home or Dining Out)

Spread bun with Dijon and mayo or avocado. Place chicken breast, spinach, onion, and tomato on bun. Enjoy with an apple. If dining out, order a 12" chicken sandwich from Subway. Save half for midafternoon. Starbucks also has a great turkey sandwich.

Nutrition facts: 395 calories, 25 grams protein, 51 grams carbohydrates, 11 grams fat

PROTEIN POWERED	3 oz grilled skinless chicken breast 1 slice of fat-free cheese (optional)
CARBOHYDRATE CONCENTRATED	1 whole wheat bun 1 medium apple or, if dining out, order 1 small lemonade
FAT FRIENDLY	Cooking spray 1 Tbsp light mayo or mashed avocado
FREE FOODS	Dijon mustard Spinach leaves Red onion Tomato Water, tea

MIDAFTERNOON
Pumpkin Pie Cottage Cheese

See Kick-Start Day 4, on page 129.

Nutrition facts: 333 calories, 23 grams protein, 49 grams carbohydrates, 8 grams fat

DINNER
Cilantro Lime Sea Bass

See recipe on page 267. Serve raspberries with agave nectar for dessert.

Nutrition facts per serving: 350 calories, 22 grams protein, 49 grams carbohydrates, 10 grams fat

PROTEIN POWERED	sea bass
CARBOHYDRATE CONCENTRATED	couscous raisins raspberries agave nectar
FAT FRIENDLY	Extra virgin olive oil
FREE FOODS	Lime juice, cilantro, ginger Water, tea

CHRISTINE'S NUTRITION NUGGETS Cilantro contains an antibacterial compound that may prove to be a natural means for fighting *Salmonella*. Pumpkin has been shown to help manage hyperglycemia and hypertension.

DAY 8

BREAKFAST

Breakfast Bagel Sandwich

See recipe on page 240.

Nutrition facts per serving: 369 calories, 27 grams protein, 44 grams carbohydrates, 9 grams fat

PROTEIN POWERED	Extra-lean turkey bacon Liquid egg whites Reduced-fat cream cheese
CARBOHYDRATE CONCENTRATED	Oat bran bagel
FAT FRIENDLY	Cooking spray Omega-3 light spread
FREE FOODS	Tomato Water, tea, coffee

LUNCH

Baked Chips and Cheesy Salsa

In a medium bowl, combine cottage cheese, olives and "free" veggies and mix well. Dip baked chips into cheesy salsa mixture and enjoy.

Nutrition facts: 357 calories, 23 grams protein, 47 grams carbohydrates, 9 grams fat

PROTEIN POWERED	$^3/_4$ c low-fat, low-sodium cottage cheese
CARBOHYDRATE CONCENTRATED	25 baked chips
FAT FRIENDLY	9 black olives, diced
FREE FOODS	$^1/_4$ c sliced scallions 1 Tbsp diced jalapeño chile peppers $^1/_4$ c diced red bell pepper Salsa Water, tea

MIDAFTERNOON
Fruity Bagel Dippers

In a medium bowl, combine all ingredients except bagel and beverage, and mix well. Dip bagel into mix. Enjoy!

Nutrition facts: 380 calories, 25 grams protein, 64 grams carbohydrates, 4 grams fat

PROTEIN POWERED	½ c low-fat, low-sodium cottage cheese
CARBOHYDRATE CONCENTRATED	1 6-oz container light yogurt Handful of blueberries 1 whole wheat bagel
FAT FRIENDLY	1 pinch slivered almonds
FREE FOODS	Water, tea

DINNER
Christine's Born-Again Lasagna

See recipe on page 262.

Nutrition facts per serving: 467 calories, 34 grams protein, 61 grams carbohydrates, 8 grams fat

PROTEIN POWERED	Extra-lean ground turkey Fat-free ricotta cheese Fat-free mozzarella cheese
CARBOHYDRATE CONCENTRATED	Whole wheat no-boil lasagna noodles Pasta sauce 1 slice whole wheat sourdough bread
FAT FRIENDLY	Extra virgin olive oil
FREE FOODS	Garlic Bell pepper Mushrooms Spices Water, tea

CHRISTINE'S NUTRITION NUGGETS Avocado is packed with vitamin E, which is great for preventing the onset of cardiovascular disease. It's also packed with soluble fiber, which helps to stabilize blood sugar.

DAY 9

BREAKFAST

Denver Omelet with Breakfast Potatoes

See recipe on page 243.

Nutrition facts per serving: 365 calories, 26 grams protein, 47 grams carbohydrates, 8 grams fat

PROTEIN POWERED	Liquid egg whites Lean Canadian bacon Fat-free milk
CARBOHYDRATE CONCENTRATED	Potato
FAT FRIENDLY	Extra virgin olive oil
FREE FOODS	Onion Green bell pepper Water, tea, coffee

LUNCH

Sandwich and Baked Chips (At Home or Dining Out)

To make at home, spread mustard and mayo on each slice of bread. Place turkey and favorite veggies into sandwich. Enjoy with 1 handful of baked chips and a pickle spear.

Nutrition facts: 434 calories, 27 grams protein, 62 grams carbohydrates, 10 grams fat

PROTEIN POWERED	3 oz or 3 slices smoked turkey
CARBOHYDRATE CONCENTRATED	10 baked chips (or 1 handful) 2 slices of whole wheat bread
FAT FRIENDLY	1 Tbsp light mayo
FREE FOODS	Dijon mustard Onion Lettuce Tomato Dill pickle spear Water, tea

MIDAFTERNOON
High-Fiber, Low-Fat Protein Bar with Anjou Pear
Grab and go!

Nutrition facts: 373 calories, 27 grams protein, 57 grams carbohydrates, 8 grams fat

PROTEIN POWERED	Low-fat, high-fiber protein bar (I like the Clif Builder's Bar)
CARBOHYDRATE CONCENTRATED	1 medium Anjou pear
FAT FRIENDLY	There is fat in the protein bar.
FREE FOODS	Water, tea

DINNER
Chicken Kebabs with Rice Pilaf (At Home or Dining Out)
To make at home, see recipe on page 273 or order at any Greek restaurant.

Nutrition facts: 377 calories, 22 grams protein, 45 grams carbohydrates, 12 grams fat

PROTEIN POWERED	2½ oz grilled skinless chicken breast
CARBOHYDRATE CONCENTRATED	½ c rice pilaf
FAT FRIENDLY	Extra virgin olive oil spray
FREE FOODS	Garlic Bell pepper Mushroom Tomato Water, tea

CHRISTINE'S NUTRITION NUGGETS Remember that you are free to cut your meal in half at any time and enjoy "free" veggies between meals. Bell peppers are one of the three Bs—broccoli, bell peppers, and Brussels sprouts—that are a good source of vitamin C.

DAY 10

BREAKFAST

Apple Raisin Oatmeal

Prepare oats according to package directions. Add raisins, apples, and cinnamon. Enjoy with a side of egg whites to keep blood sugar stable.

Nutrition facts: 349 calories, 22 grams protein, 51 grams carbohydrates, 7 grams fat

PROTEIN POWERED	4 egg whites, hard-boiled or scrambled
CARBOHYDRATE CONCENTRATED	1 c slow-cooked steel-cut oats 2 Tbsp raisins 1/2 c diced apple
FAT FRIENDLY	1 Tbsp slivered almonds
FREE FOODS	Cinnamon Sweetener such as Splenda or stevia Water, tea, coffee

LUNCH

Low-Fat Tuna Sandwich

In a medium bowl, combine tuna, egg, black olives, mayo, Dijon, relish, celery, and onion. Season with salt and pepper to taste. Place mixture onto bread slices and top with cucumber, sprouts, and tomato. Enjoy with pomegranate juice.

Nutrition facts: 395 calories, 28 grams protein, 45 grams carbohydrates, 12 grams fat

PROTEIN POWERED	2 oz chunky light tuna* 1 hard-boiled egg, diced *If pregnant, use canned chicken breast.
CARBOHYDRATE CONCENTRATED	2 slices whole wheat bread 1/4 c pomegranate juice
FAT FRIENDLY	1 Tbsp diced black olives 1 Tbsp light mayo
FREE FOODS	1 tsp Dijon mustard 1 tsp dill pickle relish Celery and onion, diced Salt and ground black pepper Cucumber, sprouts, tomato Water, tea

MIDAFTERNOON
String Cheese and Fruit
Grab and go!

Nutrition facts: 306 calories, 20 grams protein, 44 grams carbohydrates, 8 grams fat

PROTEIN POWERED	3 sticks reduced-fat string cheese
CARBOHYDRATE CONCENTRATED	1½ c red seedless grapes
FAT FRIENDLY	No need to add fat because there is fat in the string cheese.
FREE FOODS	Water, tea

DINNER
Smoked Salmon Bagel
Toast bagel and spread with cream cheese. Place salmon, olives, and "free" veggies on bagel and enjoy.

Nutrition facts: 392 calories, 32 grams protein, 58 grams carbohydrates, 5 grams fat

PROTEIN POWERED	1 slice packaged smoked salmon 2 Tbsp fat-free cream cheese
CARBOHYDRATE CONCENTRATED	Whole wheat bagel
FAT FRIENDLY	There is heart-healthy fat in the salmon.
FREE FOODS	Tomato Green onion Water, tea

CHRISTINE'S NUTRITION NUGGETS Eggs are an excellent source of biotin, a vitamin used in breaking down fat, protein, and carbs.

DAY 11

BREAKFAST

Honey Nut Apple Crunch

In a medium bowl, mix all ingredients together and enjoy.

Nutrition facts: 367 calories, 27 grams protein, 58 grams carbohydrates, 5 grams fat

PROTEIN POWERED	1 8-oz container 0% plain Greek yogurt
CARBOHYDRATE CONCENTRATED	1 large diced apple 1 Tbsp honey or agave nectar
FAT FRIENDLY	1 Tbsp crushed walnuts
FREE FOODS	Cinnamon Water, tea, coffee

LUNCH

Christine's Super Bowl Sunday Nachos

Place baked tortilla chips on a large, microwave-safe plate. Cover evenly with cheese and microwave 60 sec. Add remaining ingredients and enjoy.

Nutrition facts: 377 calories, 25 grams protein, 47 grams carbohydrates, 8 grams fat

PROTEIN POWERED	1 oz fat-free Cheddar cheese, shredded 1½ oz fat-free Monterey Jack cheese, shredded
CARBOHYDRATE CONCENTRATED	30 baked tortilla chips or 3 handfuls
FAT FRIENDLY	9 black olives, diced
FREE FOODS	¼ bell pepper ¼ c sliced scallions 1 Tbsp diced jalapeño chile peppers ¼ c diced tomato Salsa Water, tea

MIDAFTERNOON
Healthy Pizza

Preheat oven to 375ºF. Spread ½ c marinara sauce on each half of bagel. Add cheese, olives, and your favorite "free" veggies and place on a cookie sheet covered with aluminum foil. Toast in oven for 10–15 min, or until desired doneness.

Nutrition facts: 390 calories, 28 grams protein, 58 grams carbohydrates, 6 grams fat

PROTEIN POWERED	½ c shredded fat-free mozzarella cheese
CARBOHYDRATE CONCENTRATED	1 toaster-size whole wheat bagel 1 c marinara sauce
FAT FRIENDLY	5 black olives, sliced
FREE FOODS	Onion Mushrooms Bell pepper Minced garlic Water, tea

DINNER
Grilled Halibut with Quinoa and Asparagus

Preheat grill to medium heat. Brush fish with olive oil, then rub with your favorite spices. Brush asparagus spears with olive oil and sprinkle with your favorite spices. Place fish and asparagus on grill and cook until fish flakes easily. Serve with quinoa or brown rice. Finish with raspberries sweetened with agave nectar.

Nutrition facts: 360 calories, 28 grams protein, 47 grams carbohydrates, 9 grams fat

PROTEIN POWERED	3½ oz halibut, raw
CARBOHYDRATE CONCENTRATED	½ cup cooked quinoa ¾ c raspberries 2 tsp agave nectar
FAT FRIENDLY	1 tsp extra virgin olive oil
FREE FOODS	Herbs, spices Asparagus spears Water, tea

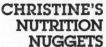 **CHRISTINE'S NUTRITION NUGGETS** Quinoa is a grain that is similar to rice, yet it offers more fiber and protein per serving. Best of all, quinoa also contains the nine essential amino acids.

DAY 12

BREAKFAST
Breakfast Bagel Sandwich

See recipe on page 240.

Nutrition facts per serving: 369 calories, 27 grams protein, 44 grams carbohydrates, 9 grams fat

PROTEIN POWERED	Extra-lean turkey bacon Liquid egg whites Reduced-fat cream cheese
CARBOHYDRATE CONCENTRATED	Oat bran bagel
FAT FRIENDLY	Cooking spray Omega-3 light spread
FREE FOODS	Tomato Salt and ground black pepper

LUNCH
Super-Fast Tuscan Polenta

Cut polenta into $\frac{1}{2}$"-thick slices. Using a spoon to partially hollow out the centers, spread polenta slices with marinara sauce. Sprinkle with cheese and microwave 1–2 min. Top with chopped basil and enjoy!

Nutrition facts: 320 calories, 25 grams protein, 50 grams carbohydrates, 2 grams fat

PROTEIN POWERED	$\frac{1}{2}$ c shredded fat-free mozzarella cheese
CARBOHYDRATE CONCENTRATED	1 oz ready-made polenta $\frac{1}{2}$ c low-fat marinara sauce
FAT FRIENDLY	Olive oil cooking spray
FREE FOODS	1 basil leaf Water, tea

MIDAFTERNOON
Deli Slices and Fruit

Combine mayo with honey mustard. Roll and dip slices into mixture. Enjoy with 2 pieces of summer fresh fruit.

Nutrition facts: 318 calories, 17 grams protein, 44 grams carbohydrates, 8 grams fat

PROTEIN POWERED	3 low-sodium deli slices (turkey, ham, or chicken)
CARBOHYDRATE CONCENTRATED	1 large peach 1 large nectarine
FAT FRIENDLY	1 Tbsp light mayo
FREE FOODS	1 Tbsp honey mustard Water, tea

DINNER
Baked Turkey, Sweet Potato, and Steamed Broccoli (At Home or Dining Out)

To make at home, roast a turkey breast or purchase premade at the grocery store. Wrap sweet potato with plastic wrap and microwave 6–7 min; remove plastic wrap and slice down the middle. Sprinkle with brown sugar. Steam broccoli with garlic salt and pepper. Add a little lemon juice. Serve and enjoy.

Nutrition facts: 398 calories, 32 grams protein, 56 grams carbohydrates, 6 grams fat

PROTEIN POWERED	3 oz roasted skinless turkey breast
CARBOHYDRATE CONCENTRATED	1 medium (6-oz) sweet potato 1 tsp brown sugar
FAT FRIENDLY	Extra virgin olive oil spray
FREE FOODS	Broccoli Garlic salt and freshly ground black pepper Lemon juice Water, tea

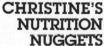 **CHRISTINE'S NUTRITION NUGGETS** The fatty acids in fish oil and olive oil not only help with the prevention of heart disease but also have an anti-inflammatory effect.

DAY 13

BREAKFAST

Chocolate Peanut Butter Smoothie

Place all ingredients into a blender and mix until consistency is smooth and creamy. Enjoy!

Nutrition facts: 335 calories, 25 grams protein, 44 grams carbohydrates, 9 grams fat

PROTEIN POWERED	1 scoop chocolate-flavored protein powder (I use Jay Robb's brand)
CARBOHYDRATE CONCENTRATED	2 small frozen bananas
FAT FRIENDLY	1 Tbsp natural peanut butter
FREE FOODS	10 ice cubes 1–2 c water Tea, coffee

LUNCH

Frozen Meal (Any brand that has approximately 1 part protein to 2 parts carbs)

Find any frozen meal that is high in protein and low in fat such as Chicken Florentine by Lean Cuisine Healthy Portions. If the carbs are too low, you can add a small piece of fruit to your meal. Then just zap and go!

PROTEIN POWERED	Chicken
CARBOHYDRATE CONCENTRATED	Carrots Pasta
FAT FRIENDLY	Most frozen meals contain fat. If not, have a serving of nuts on the side.
FREE FOODS	Water, tea

MIDAFTERNOON
Greek Yogurt with Honey and Walnuts

Combine ingredients in a medium bowl and enjoy.

Nutrition facts: 363 calories, 29 grams protein, 52 grams carbohydrates, 6 grams fat

PROTEIN POWERED	1 8-oz container 0% plain Greek yogurt
CARBOHYDRATE CONCENTRATED	$^1/_3$ c low-fat granola $^1/_4$ c blueberries 1 Tbsp honey
FAT FRIENDLY	1 Tbsp crushed walnuts
FREE FOODS	Water, tea

DINNER
Rosemary-Rubbed Salmon with Brown Rice and Steamed Artichoke

Steam artichoke over low heat for 30–40 min. Meanwhile, wash salmon with warm water and pat dry. Spray olive oil onto salmon filet. Rub with minced garlic, rosemary, salt and pepper. Squeeze a hint of lemon juice onto fish. Grill until fish flakes easily with a fork (about 4 min each side). Serve with brown rice and steamed artichoke.

Nutrition facts: 394 calories, 27 grams protein, 56 grams carbohydrates, 9 grams fat

PROTEIN POWERED	3 4 oz salmon (raw)
CARBOHYDRATE CONCENTRATED	$^3/_4$ c cooked brown rice 1 medium steamed artichoke
FAT FRIENDLY	Extra virgin olive oil spray There are heart-healthy omega-3s in the salmon fillet.
FREE FOODS	1 tsp minced garlic 1 tsp minced rosemary Salt and ground black pepper Lemon wedges Water, tea

CHRISTINE'S NUTRITION NUGGETS Artichokes contain a compound known to help cleanse the liver of toxins . . . so eat up!

DAY 14

BREAKFAST

High-Protein Cereal with Berries

Make yourself a bowl and enjoy!

Nutrition facts: 353 calories, 30 grams protein, 60 grams carbohydrates, 3 grams fat

PROTEIN POWERED	³/₄ c Kashi high-protein crunchy cereal ³/₄ c fat-free milk or soy milk
CARBOHYDRATE CONCENTRATED	Cereal should contain both carbs and protein. ¹/₂ c fresh blueberries
FAT FRIENDLY	It's in the cereal!
FREE FOODS	Water, tea, coffee

LUNCH

Sushi (Dining Out)

Order at your favorite sushi hot spot!

Nutrition facts: 326 calories, 22 grams protein, 44 grams carbohydrates, 4 grams fat

PROTEIN POWERED	2 pieces salmon roll 2 pieces tuna roll* 2 pieces yellowtail roll *If pregnant, swap tuna for salmon. See Christine's Nutrition Nugget on page 133.
CARBOHYDRATE CONCENTRATED	Sushi is wrapped in rice, thus no need to add other carbs to this meal.
FAT FRIENDLY	¹/₅ diced avocado is usually found in sushi, so no need to add more fat to this meal.
FREE FOODS	Low-sodium soy sauce Wasabi 1 c steamed veggies Water, tea

CHRISTINE'S NUTRITION NUGGETS Wasabi is a spice known for its ulcer-fighting potential. A 2004 South Korean study suggests that Japanese horseradish can kill ulcer-causing *Helicobacter pylori* bacteria.

MIDAFTERNOON
Movie Lovers' Snack

Prepare popcorn according to package directions. Grab jerky and dried apricots and watch your favorite flick!

Nutrition facts: 334 calories, 25 grams protein, 55 grams carbohydrates, 3 grams fat

PROTEIN POWERED	1¹/₂ oz turkey jerky
CARBOHYDRATE CONCENTRATED	2 c low-fat, low-sodium microwave or air-popped popcorn 8 dried apricots
FAT FRIENDLY	5 sprays of low-calorie butter spray
FREE FOODS	Water, tea

DINNER
Sicilian-Style Chicken and Rice

See recipe on page 270.

Nutrition facts per serving: 414 calories, 33 grams protein, 56 grams carbohydrates, 6 grams fat

PROTEIN POWERED	4 oz skinless chicken breast
CARBOHYDRATE CONCENTRATED	Rice Tomato sauce
FAT FRIENDLY	Extra virgin olive oil
FREE FOODS	Garlic Bell pepper Mushrooms Oregano Ground red pepper Water, tea

CHAPTER 12

Supplemental Insurance

I have always recommended that my clients take three supplements daily: a multivitamin, a B-complex supplement, and an omega-3 fatty acid supplement. As a nutritionist, I know this will prevent them from developing vitamin or mineral deficiencies, and I know the omega-3s will help combat bad fats. Clients will invariably ask me which brands I recommend, and my answer has always been the same: "Any brand."

Ironically, I haven't always followed my own recommendations. I used to feel that in order to set a good example, I should get all of my own nutrients from whole natural foods. If I ate a balanced diet from a large variety of sources, I thought, I would get 100 percent of the nutrients my body needed, right?

Wrong.

I love to cook and I use all kinds of different fresh, whole, natural ingredients. I eat many different types of proteins, and overall, I assumed that my healthy variety would provide me with all the micronutrients my body needed. But in 2005, I had my hair colored and I got a little wake-up call.

Before I knew it, my hair was brittle and broken. I would like to blame it on the colorist, but really my hair was too weak for the treatment. It was a frightening thing to see. I soon realized that my hair was not strong enough to withstand the flat iron every day, so I cut back to a few times a week. Still, my hair was coming out in clumps in the shower. It was so bad that I considered cutting it short or getting extensions or (God forbid) a wig. How did I get myself into this situation? I really thought I had been eating a great variety of foods, which should have been providing all the nutrients my hair needed. How could I be a "healthy" nutritionist with my hair breaking off? Who wants to listen to a balding woman? When your hair isn't healthy, it makes you want to crawl into a dark cocoon and hide from the world.

I learned one of those painful lessons: Vitamins and minerals are really no big deal—unless you aren't getting enough of them. I knew it was time to look into vitamin supplements.

In 1941, the United States Food and Drug Administration (FDA) developed the Recommended Daily Allowance (RDA) of essential vitamins and minerals. The purpose of the RDA was to prevent diseases caused by nutrient deficiencies. Back in those post-Depression/WWII-era days, food was often rationed. Many Americans—including my own grandparents—struggled to get enough to eat. Therefore, nutrient deficiencies were a lot more common. These days, there are a lot fewer Americans who are starving, but due to the lack of food variety, nutrient deficiencies are still relatively common.

The symptoms of vitamin deficiencies are often subtle and hard to pinpoint, and sometimes they aren't much different from the minor complaints we experience every day, such as fatigue, confusion, or emotional disturbances. Others are harder to ignore. Severe vitamin A deficiency can cause blindness (unlikely but possible), while a lack of niacin (vitamin B$_3$) can cause dementia. Those symptoms are extreme, but trust me, if you don't have the essential micronutrients you need, eventually your body will become sick.

The labels of all foods and supplements in the United States show the "% Daily Value" of vitamins and minerals based on the RDA values. The FDA revises its list every 5 or 10 years to reflect new research, but the RDAs are *minimums required to prevent disease*. Clearly my hair was telling me that even if I was taking in the minimum, it wasn't enough for vibrant health. The FDA also recommends upper limits on some of the vitamins to keep people from overdosing. You want to get enough but not too much. Here is the list of essential micronutrients. These are the vitamins and minerals for which the FDA has established a *minimum* level needed to assure good health.

VITAMINS	MINERALS
Vitamin A	Calcium
Thiamin (Vitamin B_1)	Chloride
Riboflavin (Vitamin B_2)	Chromium
Niacin (Vitamin B_3)	Copper
Pantothenic acid (Vitamin B_5)	Flouride
Vitamin B_6	Iodine
Folate (Vitamin B_9)	Iron
Vitamin B_{12}	Magnesium
Biotin	Manganese
Vitamin C	Phosphorus
Vitamin D	Potassium
Vitamin E	Selenium
Vitamin K	Sodium
	Zinc

At first I just wanted to know the vitamins that would help my hair. After dissecting the functions of each vitamin and mineral, I reached this conclusion: I needed *all* of them. When you start looking at the problems that can result from deficiencies and the benefits that come with proper nutrition, you see that every vitamin and mineral is important. Right about that point, I realized that it would be silly to take a specific set of vitamins for my hair and omit several others, possibly leading something else to go wrong. So I realized that the safest and smartest course of action was to meet all the RDAs, not just those that would specifically help my hair. You should do the same. Here are my recommendations.

Multivitamin: I recommend that all my clients take a multivitamin. However, it is important to note that some mineral compounds interfere with the absorption of others. For instance, calcium hinders iron absorption. One multivitamin might claim to have it all, from A to Zinc, but your body might not be able to use all these nutrients at once. Others include only tiny amounts of one or more nutrient, and still other multivitamin formulas exclude iron. I suggest you choose a multivitamin that contains no iron unless you have been told specifically by a doctor to take iron. My eating plan will provide plenty without overdoing it.

Use caution when considering a multivitamin that touts an "add-on" ingredient that makes it different. This "add-on" might include extracts from various herbs, roots, stems, flowers, tree bark, or other unusual sources. These other extracts are then marketed (carefully, so as not to violate the law) to deliver special benefits that are unique from those of the other multivitamins. Some of these claims are absolutely legitimate; others may not be. I am a huge fan of antioxidants in foods and supplements, so if you are going to buy a multivitamin with an add-on, look for antioxidant benefits. Antioxidants neutralize free radicals (molecules that cause cellular damage) and are thus thought to help the body combat pollutants in the environment—potentially carcinogenic ones. And they work in concert with some of the essential minerals. But even if your vitamin includes antioxidants, don't forget to eat plenty of fresh fruits (and wash them really well to get rid of any harmful residues).

B vitamins: Unlike all the mineral compounds, B vitamins often act in concert with one another rather than individually. Researchers have a hard time pinpointing the effects of one or another B vitamin because often the nutrients are interdependent. This is one of the reasons I recommend that my clients take a B-complex supplement (a supplement that contains all of the B vitamins in one) rather than a product that contains one of the B vitamins alone. In other words, don't spend your money on a bottle of niacin capsules, biotin tablets, or any other individual compound. Simply buy a B complex to include all of them at once for the best effect. B vitamins pass through the body quickly, so they need to be replenished daily. Choose a formula with no more than 1,000 percent of the US RDA of each of the B vitamin compounds—any more is unnecessary.

Omega-3 fatty acids: My other primary recommendation is an

Skinny Chick 10-Week Transformation

HUSBAND AND WIFE TESTIMONIAL

NAME: MICHELLE E.

AGE: 37

TOTAL POUNDS LOST: 27

TOTAL INCHES LOST: 37

Most women I know who went off to college put on the "freshman 15"; I put on the freshman 25. That was when I first started gaining weight. I took it off, but I put it back on again, and it's a different story when you're in your thirties as far as losing weight goes.

I've tried every single weight loss program on the market. After I got married, my husband and I both put on a ton of weight, and I couldn't shed that weight no matter what I tried. Everything just made me gain more weight. I would lose 5 or 7 pounds and then I would crash and start eating and eating. I was like a drug addict, completely out of control. I would get moody, exhausted, and collapse in the afternoon. All these failures sent me on bingeing sprees for days on end. I was very upset about it.

When I first started Christine's program, she explained blood sugar and made a diagram about how what you eat affects your blood sugar. She explained that you need a balance, including carbs. The great thing was she gave me all these carbs I *wanted* to eat. I couldn't believe the size of my breakfast and my lunch. My husband would ask, "Are you sure you can eat all that?" and I'd tell him, "That's what Christine says!" So there I was, eating all the carbs people had told me not to eat, and feeling satisfied all day long. And I never once in 10 weeks ran to the ice cream store or the doughnut shop or ate a pastry—which is a miracle for me. I never once binged, nor did I have the urge to binge. Now I feel wonderful. I feel vibrant. My body is thanking me. My husband's happy.

It's not even about vanity; it's about your health. At 37, I was already having weight-related health issues. I lived in sweatpants because that's all I could fit into. I didn't want to go to social functions. We live in Hollywood—my husband's a musician. Can you imagine being heavy and having to go into that world? It's a nightmare.

Before I started the program, I started having medical problems. I had never before felt the health consequences of being overweight, and to be feeling that way at 37 was scary. If I hadn't found this program, I can't imagine where I would be today or a year from today. I probably would be heading for an early grave.

Additional comments from Michelle's husband, Steve:

Just by eating what Michelle eats, I've lost close to 30 pounds without even trying. You stay full throughout the day. With a lot of diets, you find yourself starving and craving and crashing, and your blood sugar levels are all over the place. This is more of a lifestyle plan. You develop healthy habits almost in spite of yourself.

I wasn't planning to go on a diet. Michelle came home with this information one day, and I just jumped on board. Now our friends call us the incredible shrinking couple. And we're going to be eating this way for the rest of our lives.

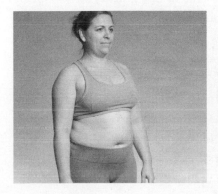
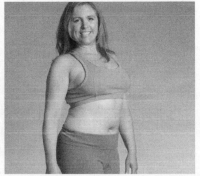

omega-3 fatty acid supplement. Omega-3s are the good fats described in Chapter 9. They can help you lose weight, improve your mood, and lower your risk of heart disease. (I also believe they help make my skin and hair look shinier and healthier, but I suppose shiny hair is less important than a heart attack!) I recommend that everybody take an omega-3 supplement with 600 milligrams eicosapentaenoic acid (EPA) and 400 milligrams docosahexaenoic acid (DHA) every day. It is best to take this in two doses. I like to have one capsule before breakfast and another before dinner, to avoid the dreaded fish burps. Make sure to buy yours from a reputable manufacturer that will provide certification of product purity if requested.

What I found out about the health supplement industry would fill another entire book. In 1994, President Clinton signed into law the Dietary Supplement Health Education Act (DSHEA) regulating label requirements. This act was intended to help consumers make informed choices about supplements. Since that time, you might have noticed that the Internet has become used widely for communication and marketing. The result? Vitamin and health supplement products have proliferated enormously, so much so that some people think vitamins are nothing but a spam scam that appears in our inboxes every day. Body part enlargement schemes aside, confusion about health supplements and weight loss products is at a nearly unimaginable level. It is impossible to keep up with the number of products on the market, and it is harder than ever simply to go out and find high-quality vitamins.

You can find all of these supplements in any grocery store or pharmacy. I know of several product manufacturers that do microbial testing of each product batch along with "assay" testing (ingredient concentration analysis by a third-party laboratory) to ensure the highest possible purity and quality. Most manufacturers do not go to such lengths, as it is not required by law as of this writing.

In order to make your life easier, I developed my own line of healthy supplements. They are up to the minute with everything you need to help you achieve optimum health. It is called the Simply Slimmer system, and it includes Simply B (B-complex), Simply MV (multivitamin), and Simply O-3 (omega-3 supplement). These are available at www. christineavanti.com.

What about Weight Loss Supplements?

Ephedra: Probably the biggest weight loss supplement to hit the market in recent memory was ephedra. Although it has been used for thousands of years, ephedra became extremely popular by the late 1990s as a dietary supplement. Tragically, it was found in the bodies of many people who died, including Minnesota Vikings lineman Korey Stringer and Baltimore Orioles pitcher Steve Bechler. Although ephedra was not specifically blamed for these deaths, both of these deaths were related to heatstroke, and ephedra is known to cause the body to overheat. The FDA banned the sale of ephedra in the United States in 2004.

Green tea extract: Most of the manufacturers who made money selling ephedra products have switched to other formulas that are based on the next best weight loss ingredient: green tea extract, known as EGCg (Epigallocatechin gallate). In a study published in the *American Journal of Clinical Nutrition*, EGCg was found to increase energy expenditure and fat oxidation in humans. This study was quite impressive because it was able to prove that EGCg—rather than the caffeine in the tea—was responsible for the increase in metabolic rate. I love drinking green tea because of its antioxidant, antimicrobial, and cholesterol-lowering activity. There are so many benefits from consuming tea that I could fill three more entire books on this single subject alone. However, I will only leave with a simple teaser: I recommend that you drink plenty of green tea. Should you take green tea extract supplements? I think they can be great; just don't expect miraculous results. It's fine to take a green tea–based supplement; just make sure it is from a good manufacturer and doesn't contain other ingredients that are harmful.

"Thermogenic" fat burners: From what I know, products that claim to be "thermogenic" are largely based on the effects of caffeine derived from herbs such as yerba maté and guaraná. These fat burners increase your core body temperature and decrease appetite. Before becoming a certified nutritionist, I tried my fair share of fat burners with very high hopes. Most of them caused my heart to race and put me in the worst mood. Another side effect I noticed was an increase in sugar cravings, because I was skipping meals. I recommend you avoid any supplement that claims to be a "fat burner." The most effective way to lose weight and burn fat is to follow the Skinny Chicks plan.

Carb blockers and fat blockers: I feel strongly that you should steer clear of any strategy that promises you can eat all you want and then alter the function of the body. You want your body to work as it is designed rather than "blocking" the intended functions using foreign substances.

Thyroid increasers and cortisol suppressants: These products lack scientific evidence to back them up. Don't use yourself as the guinea pig. Instead, increase your metabolism naturally and suppress cortisol by eating according to the Skinny Chicks plan.

Hoodia: Hoodia seems to be everywhere you look these days. It is purported to suppress the appetite; however, I want you to have a large appetite because that means your metabolism is working. I don't recommend any supplements that interfere with your body's natural systems. Therefore, I don't recommend hoodia. Hoodia is one of the ingredients flooding the supplement market from what I call the junker companies. Don't be fooled by the dramatic claims made in ads from the junkers—they are largely bogus.

Topical creams, gels, and sprays: Fat must be released from within, and what is on your skin has no bearing whatsoever on the situation. More hooey.

The bottom line is that there are no great weight loss shortcuts on the market. Drinking green tea or taking a green tea extract supplement may help a little bit, and B-complex vitamins work together to help your metabolism. But most weight loss supplements are phony baloney and don't help you lose anything except your hard-earned dollars. My best advice is to take only supplements that have credible published scientific proof of benefits. You know the old saying, "If it seems too good to be true . . . " For the most current information, please visit my Web site at www.christineavanti.com, and follow the Skinny Chicks program to get the healthiest body ever.

CHAPTER 13

Darnit, Get Your Lazy Butt on the Treadmill

As you have learned by now, I am an avid exerciser and have extensive background in and understanding of the subject of fitness. In 1990, I became a certified aerobics instructor, and I taught aerobics as a hobby for 14 years until the demands of my nutrition consulting grew too pressing. In the mid-1990s, I was certified through California State University at Hayward for personal fitness coaching, and I also have certifications in yoga, Spinning, and cardiovascular conditioning.

I developed the Skinny Chicks program so that even if you follow my eating plan and do no exercise whatsoever, your body will shed pounds of fat. Especially for people who are significantly overweight, it is hard to beat the effect of eating right. For those who are 20 pounds overweight or less, it is a little harder to shed the fat. Regardless, I recommend that everybody incorporate some kind of workout into their daily routines because besides helping you lose weight, exercise has so many other health benefits that it should be an integral part of your Skinny Chicks lifestyle.

In this chapter, you will find three different workouts for three different levels of fitness: Beginner, Intermediate, and Advanced. All three focus on the most effective movements for getting your body to ramp up its metabolism and burn body fat no matter what shape you are in.

Burning Body Fat

One of the biggest questions of the modern workout industry is which workouts cause the body to burn the most fat. There is a fat-melting workout promise on the cover of every fitness magazine every single month, yet you probably still don't know what type of exercise is really the best fat burner, do you? We all know that working out harder burns more calories, but are they calories from food, muscle, or body fat? Well, you no longer have to wonder, because I am going to tell you the answer.

Cardiovascular exercise works the heart muscle and is the only type of exercise responsible for extreme fat burning. Here's why.

There are two types of muscle fibers in our bodies:

1. **Slow twitch:** These reddish muscle fibers mainly contract during steady, prolonged exercise, such as a chit-chat walk with your best friend. Slow-twitch fiber cells are loaded with microscopic organelles called mitochondria, within which a cellular metabolic process called the Krebs Cycle takes place. The Krebs Cycle, also known as the TCA Cycle or the Citric Acid Cycle, is responsible for kick-starting the fat-burning process. Therefore, you will burn mostly fat when using slow-twitch muscle fibers.

Through research, we know that slow-twitch muscle fibers are doing most of the work when you are exercising within your target heart rate zone, anywhere between 65 and 85 percent of your maximal heart rate. (See below to calculate your target heart rate zone.)

2. **Fast twitch:** Fast-twitch muscle fibers mainly contract when intense, fast bursts of energy are needed—for example, when you need to get away from Godzilla and there is a huge rock wall in front of you! Fast -twitch muscle fibers are white because they do not contain as many of those precious little fat-burning mitochondrial organelles. Glycogen stores within muscle tissue mainly fuel fast-twitch muscle fibers. When the body uses glycogen stores for energy, muscle tissue is broken down and fat is hardly used, if it is used at all. Lance Armstrong is an excellent example of someone who focuses on training fast-twitch muscle

fibers. Lance's goal is to increase speed and strength. We can all agree that Lance Armstrong does not need to burn fat, thus he can afford to train his fast-twitch muscle fibers all he wants.

Most of us have been convinced that we must be moving fast and furiously if we want to burn fat and lose weight. But many studies, such as the one reported in the *Scandinavian Journal of Medicine and Science in Sports* in 2006, have proven that slow-twitch muscle fibers burn more fat than fast-twitch fibers. Not only that, but all of the ladies from the Skinny Chicks test group exercised in this manner, and it yielded phenomenal results. That means you don't need to be sweating profusely and gasping for breath when you exercise—you just need to exert enough energy to stay within your target heart rate zone.

Enter Your Target Heart Rate Zone

It's easy to figure out your target heart rate (THR) zone. On most treadmills and stationary bikes in a gym, there is a simple chart showing how to work within your THR zone. Ask a gym employee to show you how to use it and you are on your way. You will be amazed to discover that it really isn't a hard pace to maintain. Read a magazine, watch some trashy TV, improve your mind by reading a good book, and burn away fat at an easy-to-maintain pace. This is the pace that makes the body draw upon fat storage for energy.

If you are not using the stationary bike or the treadmill and you want to work in your THR, there are two options. One is to buy a heart rate monitor. These are available at any sporting goods store. They can be programmed to beep when you are working too fast or too slow. They are a really cool and effective product, and I highly recommend them. The other option is to use the following equation:

Subtract your age from 220. For instance, if you are 40 years old:

220   Take the number 220

- 40   subtract your age
_____

= 180   your Max Heart Rate (MHR)

Then take your MHR and multiply it by 65% and 85% to get the lower and upper limits of your THR zone.

Lower limit: multiply your MHR by 65%   180 x 65% = 117

Upper limit: multiply your MHR by 85%   180 x 85% = 153

So if you are 40 years old, your fat-burning target heart rate zone is between 117 heartbeats per minute and 153 heartbeats per minute. What I tell people to do is to look at that lower number; in this case, let's round it up to 120. This means that if your heart beats 12 times in 6 seconds, you are in your zone (there are 60 seconds in a minute, so if your heart beats 12 times in 6 seconds, it is beating 120 times in 60 seconds).

Now, how do you measure this without any equipment? Simple: You stop walking (or cycling, dancing, or whatever) and you find your pulse by placing two fingers flat on the side of your neck. When you feel your pulse, count the beats while watching a clock for 6 seconds. Then multiply the number of beats by 10. So if you counted 13 beats, you multiply by 10 to get 130. Bingo! You are well within your THR (117 to 153 in the example above).

I'll do the breakdown for you so that you can make sure to get into your minimum THR:

Age 20 to 33:   Aim for at least 13 heartbeats in 6 seconds (130 beats per minute, or BPM)

Age 34 to 46:   Aim for at least 12 heartbeats in 6 seconds (120 BPM)

Age 47 to 56:   Aim for at least 11 heartbeats in 6 seconds (110 BPM)

Age 57 to 70:   Aim for at least 10 heartbeats in 6 seconds (100 BPM)

Age 71 and up: Aim for at least 9 heartbeats in 6 seconds (90 BPM)

For more examples, pictures, and a THR calculator, please visit my Web site at www.christineavanti.com. You can also invest in a simple heart rate monitor. These are inexpensive and widely available.

Skinny Chick Chat

Dear Christine: I've heard some trainers say that you should work out first thing in the morning before breakfast. What's your opinion?

MONA B., SAN FRANCISCO

Mona: Many trainers say to work out early in the morning on an empty stomach and then to avoid eating for an hour afterward to burn as much fat as possible. I can see why this workout concept is attractive to busy individuals. The problem is that the body, having depleted Tank 1 (blood sugar) and Tank 2 (glycogen stores), is accessing muscle tissue for fuel along with body fat. There is no question that you will work off some fat. But most people who put their bodies in this kind of nutrient deficit will be working out while they have low blood sugar levels, which will cause them to overeat later in the day and reverse their gains (or in this case, losses). It would be better to have a small, balanced meal (such as low-fat Greek yogurt and a little low-fat granola) before the workout to keep the metabolism stable.

You need a workout that won't interrupt your eating plan. You need to eat a reasonable amount of a balance of nutrients at 4-hour intervals (remember your ABCs). So this means you should not work out on an empty stomach; rather, you should work out at any time during the day that doesn't interrupt your eating schedule. If you want to get your workout done early in the morning, simply grab a quick breakfast before you go.

EAT WELL, CHRISTINE

I'm not the only nutrition and fitness expert who strongly believes that exercise within your target heart rate zone is most effective for fat burning. Mark Twight, the owner of a training facility called Gym Jones in Salt Lake City, used this principle to get the cast of the movie 300 into ultra-ripped shape in 3 months through hard work and diet without any performance-enhancing drugs.

Although this concept may seem to defy logic, here's why it works: As we know, 1 gram of fat contains 9 units of energy (calories), whereas 1 gram of sugar (glucose)—which is found in muscle tissue—has only 4 units of energy. Because fat is a denser source of energy, you don't need to work as hard when you are using fat for fuel.

Don't "Dis" Your Muscles

Just because you're looking to burn fat doesn't mean you can ignore your muscles altogether. You need muscle to burn fat. Remember that a 135-pound woman with nice muscle tone is much smaller than a 135-pound woman with little muscle but a lot of fat, because the fat takes up much more space than the same weight in muscle. The best way to build muscle is through resistance training, exercises that use an opposing force to strengthen muscles. Resistance can be supplied by free weights (e.g., dumbbells), elastic bands, or even your own body weight.

You don't have to become a body builder or end up with an unnaturally muscular physique. But to look your best, you want to have a toned, lean body. Not only does that improve your appearance, it helps you lose weight as well, because muscle burns fat 24/7—even when you're resting. Your resting metabolic rate increases when your muscle mass increases. The more muscle you have, the faster your metabolism works. So you need to do some resistance training to build muscle to burn fat around the clock. Increased bone mass and density is another great perk associated with strength training.

Assuming that you are eating correctly and working out between meals, what is the best workout for burning body fat? The perfect fat-burning workout would be a combination of weight training and cardiovascular exercises, such as those listed on the following page.

Recommended Weekly Workout Schedule

My workout recommendations are broken out into three categories: Beginner, Intermediate, and Advanced. At each level, my workouts will focus your efforts on fat burning.

Beginner Workout—*For Nonactive People*

This beginning exercise plan is for people who have scarcely ever been inside a gym or who haven't worked out in more than 6 months. It allows the body to warm up slowly and get accustomed to using muscles that haven't been active for a while. It is easy and quick, yet it is very effective in getting the whole body involved and active. Remember that most of the people in the gym are not getting the benefit of a great nutrition plan like you are, so you will soon have amazing results.

If you are a total beginner, I highly recommend that you work with a personal trainer or other fitness professional the first time you do any of these exercises. Always consult with a physician if you have any doubts about your condition for exercising. When you exercise, it is important to work within the appropriate level of intensity for your health. For a beginning exerciser, the intensity level is not nearly as important as maintaining proper form. I recommend you work out at approximately 40 to 50 percent intensity. Aim to exercise within your target heart rate zone when doing cardio. If you have never worked out regularly, it is very important that you exercise for no more than 10 minutes on your first day. Here is a safe and effective exercise schedule for a beginner:

Skinny Chicks Cardiovascular Progression Chart

WEEK	DAY 1	DAY 2	DAY 3	DAY 4	DAY 5	DAY 6	DAY 7
1	10 min	15 min	20 min	25 min	30 min	Off	Off
2	30 min	30 min	30 min	30 min	30 min	Off	Off
3	30 min	35 min	35 min	35 min	35 min	Off	Off
4	35 min	35 min	35 min	35 min	35 min	Off	Off
5	35 min	35 min	Continue doing cardio a minimum of 4 days per week at 35 min per session to build up your cardiovascular endurance safely.				

The type of exercise you choose might include any of the following:

- Walking on a treadmill
- Walking outside
- Riding a stationary bike
- Swimming
- Elliptical trainer
- Stairclimber
- Rowing machine
- Low-impact aerobics (within your target heart rate zone only!)
- Spinning (within your target heart rate zone only!)
- Any other form of exercise that you enjoy and that involves the large muscles of the hips, thighs, and buttocks, such as salsa dancing, hiking, mountain biking, etc. I call this "fun" cardio.

Each cardiovascular exercise session should be performed in your target heart rate zone. In order to maximize the efficiency of your cardiovascular exercise, I highly recommend that you wear a heart rate monitor to ensure that you are exercising within your target heart rate zone at all times.

BEGINNER MUSCLE TONING AT HOME

Once you are comfortable with performing cardiovascular exercise at least four times per week for a minimum of 1 month, you can begin to incorporate some light toning exercises, such as the ones below. Having been a gym junkie for the past 18 years, I've learned which exercises benefit specific areas of the female anatomy most. So, for the Skinny Chicks workout, I have listed my favorites:

Reverse Lunge
Benefit: It lifts a sagging butt faster than any other exercise I've ever known (and I've tried them all).

Step 1: Stand in a doorway and place your hand on the door frame for balance.

Step 2: Start with both of your feet together. Step backward with one foot as far as you can. Bend both knees until the back knee almost touches the floor. It is important that your front knee be directly above your ankle joint. If your forward knee pushes past your ankle joint, you will put too much pressure on the front knee and can cause injury. Just tell yourself, your knees cannot be over your toes.

Step 3: Go back to the starting position by pressing through your front foot; focus on pushing through your heel. You should notice your glutes (butt) contracting . . . this is what you want.

Step 4: Alternate with the other leg.

Repetitions: Do a total of 20 alternating reverse lunges 3 days a week, and watch your tush get firm and lifted in no time!

Standing Calf Raise

Benefit: Nice calves that will look fantastic with a skirt and pair of high heels!

Step 1: Stand in a doorway with your feet hip-width apart, and place one hand on the door frame for balance.

Step 2: Slowly lift your heels off the floor as high as you can. Hold that position for 5 seconds, then lower back to the floor.

Repetitions: Do 3 sets of 10 reps. Don't forget to stretch out your calves afterward, by placing your toes against the wall while keeping your heel on the floor. Stretch one foot at a time, and lean forward. I often do these in the bathroom as I'm getting ready for work.

Wall or Countertop Pushup

Benefit: Lifts a sagging chest, so everything will start to look perky again.

Step 1: Standing up straight, place both hands on a wall or counter-top. Your hands should be slightly more than shoulder-width apart. Your feet should be about 1 to 2 feet away from the wall, so that you are leaning toward the wall at an angle. Bend your elbows and lean into the wall or countertop.

Step 2: Contract your midsection (core) and press yourself away from the wall or countertop until your arms are straight. Don't slouch in your lower back; stay as straight as you can.

Repetitions: Do a total of 3 sets of 10 pushups, 3 days a week.

Triceps Dip

Benefit: Gets rid of those flabby bat wings on the backs of your arms.

Step 1: Sit on the edge of your tub or a sturdy kitchen chair that won't tip over, and place your hands on either side of you, just under your butt.

Step 2: Straighten your arms and shift your body away from the edge so you can dip your butt down toward the floor. Place your feet as far away from your seat as you can, dig your heels into the floor, and point your toes to the ceiling.

Step 3: Dip your rear down by bending through your elbows, then press yourself back up. You should feel the backs of your arms contracting. The muscles contracting are your triceps (the "wing" part is called fat).

Repetitions: Do 3 sets of 10 dips, 3 times a week.

Ball or Floor Crunch

Benefit: Get back that six-pack that became a one-pack sometime between the ages of 19 and 39!

If you have a large exercise ball, you can perform "ball crunches"; if not, floor crunches work great, too.

Ball Crunch: Using a medium-size body ball, sit on top of the ball with your feet placed firmly on the floor. Next, walk your feet forward, and as you move forward, allow your rear to move forward too, so that your lower back is resting on the ball. Cross your arms over your chest, engage your lower stomach area, and crunch forward. Make sure you can feel your abs during each crunch.

Floor Crunch: Lay full length on a mat or floor with a padded surface. Slide your feet halfway up toward your body, and place your hands behind your upper neck. Crunch forward, keeping your chin up. Do not let your chin cave in to your neck; this ensures that you will be contracting your abs to lift you up. Come up one-quarter of the way, then release back to the floor. Repeat.

Repetitions: Start out slowly at 3 sets of 10 reps. You should be able to increase to 3 sets of 20 ab crunches fairly quickly.

BEGINNER CARDIO/TONING WORKOUT AT A GLANCE

Week 1—Beginner

DAY 1	DAY 2	DAY 3	DAY 4	DAY 5	DAY 6	DAY 7
Cardio and muscle toning	Cardio	Cardio and muscle toning	Off	Off	Cardio and muscle toning	Cardio

At Home Light Upper-Body Workout—Beginner

SET	MUSCLE GROUP	EXERCISE	REPS	INTENSITY	REST
1	Chest, shoulders, and back	Wall or Countertop Pushup (page 183)	10	50%	30 sec
2		Wall or Countertop Pushup	10	50%	30 sec
3		Wall or Countertop Pushup	10	50%	30 sec
4	Triceps	Triceps Dip (page 184)	10	50%	30 sec
5		Triceps Dip	10	50%	30 sec
6		Triceps Dip	10	50%	30 sec
	Total time:	About 7 min			

At Home Light Lower-Body Workout—Beginner

SET	MUSCLE GROUP	EXERCISE	REPS	INTENSITY	REST
1	Quads (fronts of your thighs), butt, hamstrings	Reverse Lunge (page 182)	20	50%	1 min
2	Calves	Standing Calf Raise (page 183)	10	50%	30 sec
3		Standing Calf Raise	10	50%	30 sec
4		Standing Calf Raise	10	50%	30 sec
5	Abs	Ball or Floor Crunch (page 184)	10	50%	30 sec
6		Crunch	15	50%	30 sec
7		Crunch	20	50%	30 sec
8		Crunch	20	50%	30 sec
	Total time:	About 30 min			

Week 2—Repeat Week 1 Schedule, but increase intensity and duration of cardio workout according to the chart on page 181.

Week 3—Repeat Week 2 Schedule, but increase intensity a little more and increase cardio time as indicated in the chart on page 181.

Intermediate Workout—*For People Who Are Comfortable in a Gym or Have Completed 3 Weeks of the Beginner Workout*

Now we are starting to get a little more serious. The equipment in the gym can be a great aid to getting in shape, but it is important that you learn how to use it properly to avoid injury. Safety first!

Before beginning the workout below, get into position and do each movement *without weights* for 15 reps. This is very important because it warms up your muscles and the joints. If you feel any strange pains while doing the movement without weights, stop immediately and seek advice from a knowledgeable personal trainer or fitness professional. *Do not* try the movement with weights if you feel pain without weights. If you did not feel any strange pains, go ahead and try the workout with very light weights (1- or 2.5-pound dumbbells for most exercises, no weights for the leg press) for the first set. In this phase, you are simply trying to get your muscles moving and stretching. During your rest, always stretch the muscles you are working out.

If you miss a workout, don't skip ahead; simply pick up where you left off.

Week 1—Intermediate

DAY 1	45 min cardio or fast walk around the neighborhood
DAY 2	Weights: 30-Minute Upper-Body Workout (page 188) 30 min cardio
DAY 3	45 min cardio or fast walk around the neighborhood
DAY 4	45 min cardio or fast walk around the neighborhood
DAY 5	Off
DAY 6	Weights: 30-Minute Lower-Body Workout (page 189) 30 min cardio
DAY 7	Off

30-Minute Upper-Body Workout—Intermediate

SET	MUSCLE GROUP	EXERCISE	REPS	INTENSITY	REST
1	Chest	Dumbbell Bench Press (page 190)	15	50%	45 sec
2		Dumbbell Bench Press	15	50%	45 sec
3		Pushup (page 190)	10–15	50%	90 sec
4	Shoulders	Seated Overhead Shoulder Press (page 190)	15	50%	45 sec
5		Seated Overhead Shoulder Press	15	50%	45 sec
6		Side Lateral Raise (page 191)	15	50%	90 sec
7	Back	Seated Machine Row (page 191)	15	50%	45 sec
8		Seated Machine Row	15	50%	45 sec
9		Lat Machine Pulldown (page 191)	15	50%	45 sec
10		Lat Machine Pulldown	15	50%	90 sec
11	Triceps	Triceps Cable Pushdown (page 192)	15	50%	45 sec
12		Triceps Cable Pushdown	15	50%	45 sec
13		Seated Dumbbell Extension (page 192)	15	50%	45 sec
14		Seated Dumbbell Extension	15	50%	90 sec
15	Biceps	Seated Dumbbell Curl (page 192)	15	50%	45 sec
16		Seated Dumbbell Curl	15	50%	45 sec
17		Standing Barbell Curl (page 193)	15	50%	45 sec
18		Standing Barbell Curl	15	50%	45 sec
	Total time:	About 30 min			

30-Minute Lower-Body Workout—Intermediate

SET	MUSCLE GROUP	EXERCISE	REPS	INTENSITY	REST
1		Leg Press (page 194)	20	50%	1 min
2	Quads	Leg Press	20	50%	1 min
3		Leg Press	20	50%	2 min
4		Dumbbell Reverse Lunge (page 194)	16	50%	1 min
5	Butt	Dumbbell Reverse Lunge	16	50%	1 min
6		Dumbbell Reverse Lunge	16	50%	2 min
7		Lying Leg Curl (page 194)	20	50%	45 sec
8	Hamstrings	Lying Leg Curl	20	50%	45 sec
9		Lying Leg Curl	20	50%	45 sec
10		Calf Raise (page 195)	20	50%	45 sec
11	Calves	Calf Raise	20	50%	2 min
12		Ball or Floor Crunch (page 195)	20	50%	45 sec
13	Abs	Crunch	20	50%	45 sec
14		Crunch	20	50%	45 sec
15		Crunch	20	50%	45 sec
	Total time:	About 30 min			

Week 2—Repeat Week 1 Schedule, but increase intensity in the gym to 60 percent maximum effort.

Week 3—Repeat Week 2 Schedule, but increase intensity in the gym to 70 percent maximum effort and increase fun cardio or walking on Tuesday and Saturday to 45 minutes.

INTERMEDIATE AND ADVANCED EXERCISES

Dumbbell Bench Press

Benefits: Strengthens your chest, shoulders, and triceps.

Step 1: Grab a dumbbell in each hand, lie flat on a bench with your feet flat on the floor, and tilt your pelvis forward so that each of your vertebrae are touching the bench. (If you cannot feel each of your vertebrae touching the bench, it is okay to place your feet on the bench instead of the floor. However, the first position is the safest.)

Step 2: Contract your abdominal muscles inward (this ensures a strong core). Next, press the dumbbells upward with your elbows at your sides, until your arms are extended.

Step 3: Lower the weights to the sides of your upper chest until you feel a slight stretch in your chest or shoulders. Repeat.

Pushup

Benefits: Strengthens your chest, anterior deltoids, and triceps.

Step 1: Kneel on all fours with your wrists directly under shoulders, your arms straight, and your knees under your hips. Move your hands slightly farther apart than shoulder width and tuck your hips forward so your torso forms a straight line from your head to your knees.

Step 2: Bend your elbows and lower your body toward the floor until your elbows are aligned with your shoulders.

Step 3: Push up to the starting position and repeat.

Seated Overhead Shoulder Press

Benefit: Strengthens your deltoids (shoulder muscles).

Step 1: Sit on a 90-degree-angle, back-supported bench, and grab two dumbbells. Bring the dumbbells up to the fronts of your shoulders, with your palms forward and your abs tight for a strong core.

Step 2: Press the dumbbells up and overhead in an arch motion and softly tap the dumbbells at the top.

Step 3: Lower the dumbbells slowly and repeat.

Side Lateral Raise

Benefit: Strengthens your medial deltoids (the middle muscle of your shoulders).

Step 1: Stand with your knees slightly bent and tighten your abdominals. Hold the dumbbells at your sides with your palms facing your thighs.

Step 2: Slowly raise your arms out laterally from your sides. Focus on lifting through your elbows rather than your hands (this will cause you to contract your medial deltoids more), and pause when the dumbbells are at shoulder height.

Step 3: Slowly lower the dumbbells and repeat.

Seated Machine Row

Benefits: Strengthens your back and biceps.

Step 1: Sit at a cable row machine with a small triangle handle attached to the cable. Place your feet firmly on the foot dock, grasp the handle with both hands, and slowly sit up with your back straight and your shoulders back in their sockets.

Step 2: Next, pull or row the handle in to your abs, moving your elbows as far back as possible.

Step 3: Slowly release to return the handle to the starting position, and repeat.

Lat Machine Pulldown

Benefits: Strengthens your latissimus dorsi (back muscles) and biceps.

Step 1: Sit at a pulldown machine with your legs snugly under the kneepads. With your feet firmly on the floor, grasp the wide bar with an overhand grip. Your hands should be twice your shoulder width apart (as wide as possible).

Step 2: Slightly arch your back as you pull the bar down to the top of your chest.

Step 3: Focus on keeping your elbows below the bar, pause and contract your back muscles, and slowly raise the bar back to the starting position. Do not lean back using your body weight to pull the bar down. If you notice that you are doing this, lighten the weight.

Triceps Cable Pushdown

Benefit: Strengthens your triceps.

Step 1: Stand facing a high cable pulley with your knees slightly bent, your shoulders back in their sockets, your chest forward, your elbows in line with your shoulders close to your rib cage, and your arms bent.

Step 2: Straighten your arms, pressing down toward your thighs.

Step 3: Keeping your elbows close to your rib cage, bend your arms upward and repeat.

Seated Dumbbell Extension (a.k.a. French Press)

Benefit: Strengthens your triceps.

Step 1: Start with a dumbbell weight that you can hold above your head using two hands. Sit on a bench with your back straight, your feet firmly on the floor, and your abs tight.

Step 2: Grasp the dumbbell underhand around the shaft with both hands for a firm grip, and press it above your head, contracting the backs of your arms.

Step 3: Lower slowly and repeat.

Seated Dumbbell Curl

Benefit: Strengthens your biceps.

Step 1: Sit on a 90-degree-angle, back-supported bench, and grab two dumbbells. With both feet firmly on the floor and your abs tight, hold the dumbbells using an underhand grip.

Step 2: Starting in the down position, keep your elbows close to your rib cage, bend at the elbows, and curl the weights up to the fronts of your shoulders.

Step 3: Lower slowly and repeat.

Standing Barbell Curl

Benefit: Strengthens your biceps.

Step 1: Stand straight with your shoulders back and your knees slightly bent. Grab a barbell using an underhand grip.

Step 2: Starting with the barbell in front of your thighs in the down position, keep your elbows close to your rib cage, bend at the elbows, and curl the weights up. The barbell should stay close to your body as it travels upward to the fronts of your shoulders.

Step 3: Lower slowly and repeat.

Incline Dumbbell Fly

Benefit: Strengthens your inner pectoral muscles (they make a beautiful line down the middle of the chest).

Step 1: Lie on an incline bench angled at 60 degrees, with your feet firmly on the floor and your abs tight. Hold a dumbbell in each hand above your chest. Your arms should be straight, and your palms should mirror each other.

Step 2: Next, bend your elbows out and down to align the dumbbells with your shoulders.

Step 3: Lift up and repeat.

Incline Dumbbell Press

Benefit: Strengthens your pectoral muscles.

Step 1: Lie on an incline bench angled at 60 degrees, with your feet firmly on the floor and your abs tight. Hold a dumbbell in each hand above your chest, with your arms straight and your palms facing away from your body.

Step 2: Next, bend your elbows downward until the dumbbells are aligned with your shoulders.

Step 3: Press up and lightly tap the dumbbells together upon extension. Repeat.

Leg Press

Benefits: Strengthens your quadriceps, hamstrings, and gluteal muscles.

Step 1: Sit on a 45-degree-angled leg press machine (most gyms have these), and place your feet on the platform, hip-width apart.

Step 2: Press the platform up, release the dock safety lever, and grasp the side handles. Now lower the sled by bending your knees until they are slightly beyond a 90-degree angle.

Step 3: Press up to the starting position, and focus on pressing through your heels as opposed to the balls of your feet. This helps to even the work between your quads, hamstrings, and glutes. Repeat.

Dumbbell Reverse Lunge

Benefits: Strengthens your gluteal muscles, quads, and hamstrings.

Step 1: Stand with your feet hip-width apart and grab a dumbbell in each hand. Let the dumbbells hang down at your sides, near your outer thighs.

Step 2: Begin by stepping one foot back behind you. Reach your foot back as far as you can. You should feel a stretch in the hip flexor muscle of your back leg.

Step 3: Lower yourself slowly, stopping just before your back knee touches the floor. Bring your back foot forward and repeat with the other leg.

Lying Leg Curl (a.k.a. Hamstring Curl)

Benefits: Strengthens your hamstrings and glutes.

Step 1: On a hamstring machine (found at most gyms), lie on your stomach, hook your feet under the circular ankle pad, and flex your feet (do not point your toes).

Step 2: Slowly curl your legs up and in toward your butt in an arching motion.

Step 3: Squeeze your hamstrings and glutes, then slowly release back to the starting position. Repeat.

Calf Raise

Benefit: Strengthens your calf muscles.

Step 1: Grab a dumbbell in each hand and let them hang at your sides. Stand with your feet hip-width apart and your knees slightly bent.

Step 2: Slowly lift your heels off the floor as high as you can.

Step 3: Hold the position for 5 seconds, then lower your heels back to the floor. Repeat.

Ball Crunch

Benefit: Strengthens your abs.

Step 1: Using a medium-size body ball, sit on top of the ball with your feet placed firmly on the floor.

Step 2: Next, walk your feet forward, and as you move forward, allow your rear to move forward too, so that your lower back is resting on the ball.

Step 3: Cross your arms over your chest, engage your lower stomach area, and crunch forward. Make sure you can feel your abs during each crunch.

Floor Crunch

Benefit: Strengthens your abs.

Step 1: Lay full length on a mat or floor with a padded surface. Slide your feet halfway up toward your body, and place your hands behind your upper neck.

Step 2: Crunch forward, keeping your chin up. Do not let your chin cave in to your neck; this ensures that you will be contracting your abs to lift you up.

Step 3: Come up one-quarter of the way, then release back to the floor. Repeat.

Skinny Chicks
Workout Guidelines

- Do cardio in your target heart rate zone (not too fast).

- Find an activity that you love to do— your fun cardio.

- Do your fun cardio immediately after weight training to better access body fat for energy.

- Do weight training or other resistance training to increase muscle tone. You will burn calories (and fat) during the workout and throughout the day.

- If you are just beginning, have a personal trainer or fitness professional demonstrate the exercises and machinery for you.

- Work your way gradually from very light weights to heavier weights to increase your intensity.

- Always stretch the muscles you are working between sets.

- After a few weeks, you should strive to reach 100 percent maximum exertion in your weight lifting workouts, but keep your fun cardio within your THR zone.

Advanced Workout— *For Active People or Beginners Who Have Completed 4 Weeks of the Intermediate Plan*

The next stage is for people who are ready to step it up to a level that begins to reshape the body. By now you should have figured out some options for your cardio. You've also warmed up your muscles and joints so that weight training can be increased. You only have to work out 3 days per week, but I have stacked the workouts so that you are getting the maximum fat burning benefit. If you like, you may do the cardio on the off days to better fit your schedule, but it is best to do it as a continuous block to access the most fat storage for energy. Try to do the entire routine at least once on the weekend when you have more time.

Week 2 is identical to Week 1 except that the upper- and lower-body weight training circuits are alternated. If you look at the table beginning on page 198, you'll see that on the first set of each new muscle group, the intensity is always 50 percent, meaning that you should be able to perform the exercise with a bit of strain . . . but not zero strain. This is just a "warmup" set to get your muscles and joints prepared for the heavy workload to come in the next set, and it uses a light weight and more reps. As the weeks go on and you grow more comfortable with your weights, increase the intensity of your last set for each muscle group by grabbing a slightly heavier weight. As an alternative to doing the workout, you may do a body sculpting class.

Week 1—Advanced

DAY 1	DAY 2	DAY 3	DAY 4	DAY 5	DAY 6	DAY 7
Weights: 45-Minute Lower-Body Workout (page 189) at 85% of maximum effort		Weights: 45-Minute Upper-Body Workout (page 188) at 85% max effort		Off	Weights: 45-Minute Lower-Body Workout at 85% max effort	
30–60 min of cardio	1 hr cardio	1 hr cardio	30–60 min of cardio		1 hr cardio immediately after gym	1 hr cardio

Week 2—Advanced

DAY 1	DAY 2	DAY 3	DAY 4	DAY 5	DAY 6	DAY 7
Weights: 45-Minute Lower-Body and Abs Workout at 85% of max effort	Off	Weights: 45-Minute Upper-Body Workout at 85% of max effort	Off	Off	Weights: 45-Minute Lower-Body and Abs Workout at 85% of max effort	Off
1 hr fun cardio—do immediately after gym or tomorrow		1 hr fun cardio—do immediately after gym or tomorrow			1–2 hrs fun cardio immediately after gym	

45-Minute Upper-Body Workout—Advanced

SET	MUSCLE GROUP	EXERCISE	REPS	INTENSITY	REST
1		Dumbbell Bench Press (page 190)	20	50%	45 sec
2		Dumbbell Bench Press	12	85%	45 sec
3	Chest	Dumbbell Bench Press	12	85%	45 sec
4		Incline Dumbbell Fly (page 193)	12	85%	45 sec
5		Incline Dumbbell Fly	10	85–100%	90 sec
6		Seated Overhead Shoulder Press (page 190)	20	50%	45 sec
7		Incline Dumbbell Press (page 193)	12	85%	45 sec
8	Shoulders	Incline Dumbbell Press	12	85%	45 sec
9		Side Lateral Raise (page 191)	12	85%	45 sec
10		Side Lateral Raise	10	85–100%	90 sec
11		Seated Machine Row (page 191)	20	50%	45 sec
12		Seated Machine Row	15	85%	45 sec
13	Back	Seated Machine Row	15	85%	45 sec
14		Lat Machine Pulldown (page 191)	15	85%	45 sec
15		Lat Machine Pulldown	12	85–100%	90 sec

SET	MUSCLE GROUP	EXERCISE	REPS	INTENSITY	REST
16		Triceps Cable Pushdown (page 192)	20	50%	45 sec
17		Triceps Cable Pushdown	15	85%	45 sec
18	Triceps	Seated Dumbbell Extension (page 192)	15	85%	45 sec
19		Seated Dumbbell Extension	15	85%	45 sec
20		Seated Dumbbell Extension	12	85–100%	90 sec
21		Seated Dumbbell Curl (page 192)	15	50%	45 sec
22		Seated Dumbbell Curl	15	85%	45 sec
23	Biceps	Standing Barbell Curl (page 193)	15	85%	45 sec
24		Standing Barbell Curl	15	85%	45 sec
25		Standing Barbell Curl	12	85–100%	
	Total time:	About 30–40 min			

45-Minute Lower-Body and Abs Workout—Advanced

SET	MUSCLE GROUP	EXERCISE	REPS	INTENSITY	REST
1		Leg Press (page 194)	30	50%	1 min
2	Quads	Leg Press	20	85%	1 min
3		Leg Press	15	85–100%	2 min
4		Dumbbell Reverse Lunge (page 194)	20	50%	1 min
5	Butt	Dumbbell Reverse Lunge	16	85%	1 min
6		Dumbbell Reverse Lunge	16	85%	1 min
7		Lying Leg Curl (page 194)	25	50%	1 min
8	Hamstrings	Lying Leg Curl	16	85%	1 min
9		Lying Leg Curl	12	85–100%	2 min
10	Calves	Calf Raise (page 195)	20	85%	1 min
11		Calf Raise	20	85–100%	1 min

(continued)

45-Minute Lower-Body and Abs Workout—Advanced (cont.)

SET	MUSCLE GROUP	EXERCISE	REPS	INTENSITY	REST
12		Ball Crunch (page 195)	20	85%	1 min
13		Ball Crunch	20	85%	1 min
14	Abs	Ball Crunch	20	85–100%	1 min
15		Floor Crunch (page 195)	20	85%	1 min
16		Floor Crunch	20	85%	1 min
17		Floor Crunch	20	85–100%	1 min
	Total time:	About 30–40 min			

Weeks 3 and 4—Repeat Weeks 1 and 2 but gradually increase intensity level.

Don't forget to keep your body well fueled for your workouts to get the most from your time in the gym. If you are eating according to the Skinny Chicks plan, your body should have all the nutrients it needs for energy. But on days when you are not feeling 100 percent, I recommend taking a B vitamin–based energy boost before your workout (my favorite is Simply enerG, available at www.christineavanti.com).

Skinny Chick 10-Week Transformation

NAME: CASEY F.

AGE: 47

TOTAL POUNDS LOST: 17

TOTAL INCHES LOST: 21

I remember being body conscious as far back as the sixth grade. I was very involved in sports and had a muscular build. I joined the cheerleading squad, but as soon as I put that little skirt on, I felt different from the others. I wished I had skinny little legs like they did.

My involvement in sports grew throughout my teenage years, and I began to embrace my muscular build. I always managed to make working out a priority. When I entered college, I became very interested in health food—I actually became kind of fanatical about it—and I was compulsive about everything I ate. I managed to stay a size 0 until my first child was born, when I was 35, but I found it very difficult to lose the weight once the baby was born.

From that point on, things began to change. Life got in the way, and it wasn't all about me anymore. My workouts became sporadic at best; my eating habits changed. I was practically starving myself. I began to skip meals and eat foods that were higher in fats and calories. And then I found the Skinny Chicks program. Since following Christine's guidelines, I have changed from head to toe. My face is thinner and looks much younger. I have a flatter stomach and my love handles are gone. My legs are thinner and don't rub together when I walk anymore. But the greatest impact has been on my energy level. I used to go to bed exhausted, sleep for 8 hours, and wake up exhausted. Now I pop out of bed and feel great. I embrace each day and I am much more productive.

PART IV

SKINNY CHICKS

IN THE

REAL WORLD

CHAPTER 14

Skinny Chicks Have Their Ups and Downs

Here is something you might want to know. Once you have settled into your eating plan and your blood sugar levels have stabilized (anywhere from 3 days to a few weeks into your plan), your body will begin to burn fat steadily. Nearly every one of my clients tells me they feel better than they have in years, with calm, steady energy and a healthy appetite. Once you eat on my plan for a while, you get very addicted to having a consistent, stable energy level, and it will be very apparent when you don't eat right. A single massive sugar binge can upset your metabolism and blood sugar stability for several days. If, one night, you decide to throw it all to the wind and have a psycho pecan pie pig-out, you might feel lethargic for the next few days and have no desire to eat on your schedule. When there is something tough going on in your life, like a breakup or a work deadline, you may find it hard to resist saying "the heck with it" and just eat pizza and ice cream all weekend.

What many people do after a binge is make up for it by trying to eat as little as possible the next day. They revert to old fad diets and doubt the validity of real nutritional science: the ABCs. Somewhere in the back of their minds, they still hold on to the belief that the *real* way to lose weight is either to starve themselves or to avoid all carbs. But all this does is slow your metabolism, deprive your body of required nutrients, and set you up for another binge—just as holding your breath underwater sets you up to pop to the surface for air. You can't hold your breath forever, and you can't forever deny your body the nutrients it needs either. This is why it is so important to head this situation off at the pass in the first place, by avoiding major binges. And if you do have one, get up the next day and get right back on your plan.

When a client comes to my office, she may appear composed and confident. On the inside, though, most folks who walk through my door are at their wits' end. They are overwhelmed with frustration and sick of trying to lose weight and failing. During their program, I weigh them every week. I also measure body fat so I can tell them when they are gaining muscle and losing fat, even if there's no change in the number on the scale. Even so, people get incredibly discouraged when the number on the scale doesn't change or even goes up. Some people are inconsolable, and quite often, the tears just start to flow. These clients want so badly to prove that they are not a failure in my eyes and in their own hearts. The numbers on the scale seem to seal their fates as losers, but *this is simply not the case.*

There are three things to know here. The first is that no one is ever a loser for trying; the second is that eating healthfully will feed muscle and burn fat. Some people don't immediately show weight loss because they are gaining muscle while losing body fat. Bear in mind, though, that a pound of muscle is much more attractive than a pound of fat. If you have swapped a pound of muscle for a pound of fat, you have made a big improvement in your appearance already.

The third thing to know is that you are not alone. I have been around some of the world's top fitness models and competitors, and these professionals have "flat" weeks or "up" weeks as well. They may lose 6 pounds one week, then gain back a few and at other times lose only a single pound in a week. The thing to realize is that it is a normal part of the weight loss process. Eventually the weight comes off. So don't be deceived or discouraged by the scale. And don't weigh yourself more often than once a week.

It's important to realize that the more quickly weight is lost, the more likely it is that the loss is coming from water and muscle, *not* fat. If you are losing a pound or two per week, that is actually a healthy pace. And don't forget that it is *very* hard to see weight loss on yourself, because you look at yourself in the mirror every day. Somebody who hasn't seen you for a month is likely to compliment you on your weight loss even if you can't see it yet. Don't let your own mind deceive you.

More often than not, you will notice first that your clothes fit differently and that you can once again wear the jeans and tops that have been pushed to the back of your closet. There is nothing like the feeling of being able to button a button or zip a zipper that wouldn't close only a few weeks earlier.

The chart below shows the progress of three women from the Skinny Chicks 10-week test group whose weight went up and back down. Each had up weeks and down weeks as well as temporary plateaus. This is a natural part of the weight loss process. Our bodies are constantly going through metabolic and hormonal changes; we shouldn't ever be discouraged by a small increase in weight.

3 TYPICAL EXAMPLES FROM SKINNY CHICKS TEST GROUP

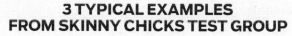

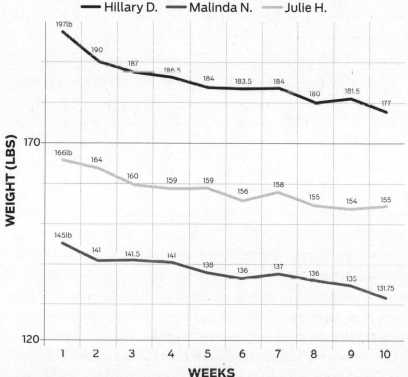

Skinny Chick 10-Week Transformation

NAME: COURTNEY H.

AGE: 20

TOTAL POUNDS LOST: 15

TOTAL INCHES LOST: 24.75

I have been overweight all my life. My mom is big, my sister is big, my brother is big—we just have big genes. When I was in middle school, I became very sick, and I had severe stomach pains for almost a year. Eventually, I was diagnosed with Crohn's disease. Once I was put on medication, including steroids, the pounds just piled on.

My dad was a single father. He was great, but he didn't have time or know how to give us the most nutritional meals. I got in the habit of eating fast foods and anything that was quick and easy, so I just kept gaining weight.

I moved to California for college and started to get sick again. In 2007, part of my intestine was removed. Even then, I still clung to my bad eating habits. I couldn't find a weight loss plan I could stick to or that would give me any results. I was getting depressed and desperate.

When I started the Skinny Chicks program, I was sure it was just going to be something else I'd try for a week and then drop. But it wasn't like that at all. The program has made me take a good look at myself and my life. I've had to face my demons and let go of things that were holding me back. Now I feel like I'm on the track to success. Christine not only taught me to eat healthfully and helped me lose weight; she also made me believe that my thoughts and words could become my reality.

As you can see, a small gain in a week is a normal part of every successful weight loss process. In this chart, all three women had two "up" weeks, but eventually they lost anywhere from 11 to 20 pounds.

Sometimes clients who have been through dieting extremes will gain a few pounds in the early days of starting my program. I can recall one example of this with a very popular celebrity client whom I'll call Susan. Susan started my program with dedication and excitement, especially when she found out that eating carbs actually helps to achieve a sleek, lean body. However, our first 2 weeks of working together were quite a challenge. Five days after starting, I received a frantic call from Susan's assistant telling me that Susan had gained 4 pounds and was literally freaking out because she had to be on camera that afternoon for a TV interview. This might sound like no big deal, but for a celebrity, 4 pounds can seem like a career killer—something that can undermine her entire family's livelihood. I advised the assistant to keep Susan calm, and to have the wardrobe stylist find her the nicest-looking long-sleeve shirt or jacket for the interview, as the first place her weight always showed was her arms. I also asked to see her in my office as soon as possible. When I finally met with Susan, I could see she was retaining a lot of water—possibly a reaction to suddenly eating carbs again. Now, bear in mind that this is a beautiful and famous woman who had previously been avoiding all carbs with the exception of a sugar binge here and there. (Oh, how I understood her issues—they hit very close to home!) I had forewarned her about this, and I reminded her that for every gram of sugar the body receives, it can hold approximately 4 grams of water. Like many low-carb zealots, Susan probably thought I was full of it, but she stuck with the plan because a friend of hers had lost 16 pounds in 1 month on my program. Thank goodness she did stick with it, because by the following week, the extra 4 pounds were gone and she went on to achieve dramatic results, losing a total of 7 percent body fat in 12 weeks. Susan continues to follow my program to this day.

So, if the scale goes up a little, don't worry about it. Not only is it a natural progression, but it might even mean you're gaining muscle. Stick it out. This program works because it's not a diet. It's the real deal for real people in real life.

CHAPTER 15

Every Day Is a Splurge Day

What if I told you that you could be a Skinny Chick and still enjoy the foods you like and eat out without guilt? It *is* possible to strike a balance between enjoying the foods you love and living your healthiest life.

A lot of diets encourage you to have a "splurge day" as part of the program. Sadly, that perpetuates the attitude that a diet is a temporary restrictive program that you can go off of when you're "done." My response to that philosophy is: *We've been splurging our entire lives, which is how we ended up gaining weight in the first place!* Enough with the splurge days; we are real people living in a real world . . . it's time to tune in to reality. We need to pull the plug on splurge days and diets altogether.

The Skinny Chicks program is not temporary or restrictive—it's a way of eating your whole life long so that you won't need a splurge day. Make room in your daily meals for a chocolate chip cookie once in a while or a slice of birthday cake like those sassy Skinny Chicks you know. (After all, why should they get to prance around with a dessert at a dinner party, while you sit there with a bottled water repeating, "No thanks, I'm on a diet, I have to wait till my 'splurge day.'") Stop dieting, stop with the splurge days, and start living. I will cheer you on and guide you every step of the way. If a food-obsessed girl like me can actually break away from the bondage of 24-hour sugar cravings, so can you.

The Sweetest Things

By now I hope you have an understanding of the insanity that once surrounded my own eating habits. The core of that insanity was my intense love of sweets. They aren't called sweets for nothing; for me, they made my sour existence tolerable. Why? Because for a brief moment, they were the only thing that anesthetized my sorrow. I remember talking with girlfriends literally for hours—not about guys or careers, but about *sweets!* I was never into drugs, but my cravings for sweets were so acute and powerful that I might as well have been a street addict.

Nevertheless, my addiction to sweet things was an integral part of what made me pursue a career in nutrition. And that led to this amazing discovery:

If you have a lean protein in your meal, you can choose whatever type of carbohydrate you wish.

The operative word here is *choose*. You can have *any* carbohydrate you want. That doesn't mean you can have *every* carbohydrate you want all at the same time. And most importantly, it must be part of a PC Combo. For example, if you are attending a wedding and they are serving grilled fish, green beans, roasted potatoes, dinner rolls, and cake, simply skip the carbs in the meal (potatoes and dinner rolls—the green beans are a free food) and count a small piece of wedding cake as the carbohydrate component of your PC Combo. Just be sure to eat your dessert within 1 hour of eating your meal. You want the sugar from the dessert to be slowed down by the amino acids from the protein in the meal. All the meals in my program are designed so that you can easily eliminate the carbs and fats and swap them for your favorite dessert.

Can you do this at every meal and still lose weight? It's possible, although I wouldn't advise it. I had a client a few years back who told me in our first appointment that she would follow my program to the letter as long as she could eat sweets with every meal. Sounds a little strange to pay a nutritionist to help with weight loss yet demand that your nutritionist allow you to eat sweets. But hey, I've been there myself, so I could relate. I advised her to find low-fat sweets with less than 50 grams of carbohydrates, and I told her that as long as she ate them along with a lean protein, she could have her cake and eat it too! That particular client lost 25 pounds in 12 weeks, and even I was amazed. I don't recommend that

The Real Skinny about Dark Chocolate

One thing some of my successful clients do is have one small piece of dark chocolate (no more than 1 ounce) after a healthy PC Combo meal. If you're going to choose a sweet treat, this is your best choice, as recent studies have shown that dark chocolate is actually good for your health. Dark chocolate contains flavonoids, antioxidants that help fight damage caused by free radicals. It also has heart health benefits, including helping to reduce high blood pressure and lower cholesterol. Look for dark chocolate (not milk or white chocolate) that has at least 70 percent or higher cocoa content. Whatever your sweet preference may be, I encourage you to feel free to have the occasional treat rather than be bound to the "diet/deprivation" mind-set. Just use your good judgment and keep eating PC Combos.

you make this a steady habit, because obviously, sweets lack protein, fiber, vitamins, minerals, and antioxidants. But that client's results show that having a dessert once in a while won't hurt or impede your progress. The Skinny Chicks program is about living and eating in the real world.

All my clients want to find ways to get their sweets, and so do I. However, consider the following: A single piece of cheesecake from The Cheesecake Factory can have as many as 1,600 calories. A large serving at Coldstone Creamery or a pint of Ben & Jerry's can easily contain more than 1,200 calories. To put that in perspective, a healthy 130-pound woman requires around 1,500 to 1,800 calories per day to maintain her body weight. Not only that, but these desserts are extremely high in saturated fats and cholesterol. Frequent trips to the ice cream parlor are not a healthy habit. So what should a sweet-toothed Skinny Chick do?

Most dieters experience a "cave-in" and eat a huge amount of sweets after trying to deprive themselves of food for a long period. So the first thing to do is eat on a regular basis in order to stabilize your blood sugar.

Once their blood sugar has been stable for 3 days or so, most of my clients find they are far less tempted to splurge.

But, if you're really jonesin' for that chocolate blackout cake (hey, just because I'm a nutritionist doesn't mean I don't enjoy rich desserts!), have a small serving, enjoy it, and move on. If you continue to resist, you are going to drive yourself bananas (or more likely, banana splits!)

The 100-Calorie Slippery Slope

Have you been to the supermarket lately? Next time you go, take a trip down the cookie aisle. Those savvy marketers are at it again. They know we're all concerned about our weight, and they know we all still want those sweets. So what have they done? They've packaged everything from Pringles to Oreos, from crackers to pretzels and nuts, in 100-calorie snack packs. The idea is that because we could never buy a bag of Oreos and eat just one or two (our blood sugar levels have us on "binge mode"), they've shrunk them into 100-calorie portions for us. Sounds like a good idea, no?

There are a number of problems with this. For one thing, you're paying top dollar for those pint-size treats. Take pretzels, for instance. If you buy a larger bag of pretzels, you may pay about 17 cents an ounce. When you buy a 100-calorie pack, you're going to pay around 40 cents an ounce—more than double the cost. And you're not getting much nutrition, either, so you're just going to be hungry later and will probably eat more than you should. You're paying twice as much for a snack that will fill you up only half as much as a better choice, such as a piece of string cheese or some yogurt and granola.

But that's not my main beef with these tiny snacklets. If I want a piece of pecan pie for dessert, I won't be satisfied with a child-size handful of cookies or chips. I'll eat the snack pack and still feel deprived. That voice inside my head will still be screaming, *I want my pecan pie!* Which means I'll probably finish off my 100-calorie treat in the blink of an eye, and before I know it, I'll have another and another . . . until I've consumed a whole meal's worth of calories. And I'll still be craving pecan pie.

So, I say, forget about the snack packs and go for the pie. Have a lean protein for dinner, have some veggies from the free food list (Appendix), and follow it up with a small piece of the pie you've been salivating over for days. When you follow the Skinny Chicks PC Combo plan, one piece will do it for you. You will satisfy your sweet tooth without having to eat the whole pie. You won't want the whole pie because you will be eating so much and so often on this program.

Artificial Sweeteners: The Good, the Bad, and the Deadly!

Although it would be great if everything we ate were made of the purest, most natural ingredients, that is not always the case. For those of us watching our weight and wanting to splurge without adding extra calories, foods made with artificial sweeteners are often the answer.

They are calorie-free and they don't spike blood sugar. So what's the problem with artificial sweeteners? Well, no one is really sure, and that could be a problem. Personally, I am neutral on the subject, although I believe some sugar alternatives are better than others. It is important to consume all things in moderation. As you follow my Skinny Chicks nutrition program, your desire for sweets will begin to diminish, and the idea of adding sweetener to your beverages and meals may lose its appeal. The great thing about this program is that you will no longer be a slave to sugar. But I could not write a nutrition book without providing a little background information, so here's the skinny on sweeteners.

All artificial sweeteners are made of different blends of molecules that trick our tastebuds into believing that they taste something sweet. Artificial sweeteners trigger the same taste receptors as sugar does. The difference is, it only takes a tiny amount of artificial sweetener to get your tongue thinking you just consumed a large amount of sugar. Artificial sweeteners are hundreds or, in some cases, even tens of thousands of times sweeter than real sugar. For example, there are 10 teaspoons of sugar in one can of Coke, while there is less than a tenth of a teaspoon of aspartame in a Diet Coke. Because artificial sweeteners work so well in such small amounts, they add almost no calories to foods and beverages while offering the same or even a higher level of sweetness.

Although the evidence on whether artificial sweeteners are harmful to human beings is inconclusive, I strongly recommend that you use them with caution. In my experience, the overuse of artificial sweeteners can cause sugar cravings. I've witnessed clients suffering from extreme sugar cravings only to find out that they use an average of 30 to 40 packets of artificial sweetener daily. I myself can recall using 10 packets of Equal while spooning half a jar of peanut butter into my mouth. Here are some of the most common sugar alternatives.

Aspartame: Commonly known as Equal. In 1996, scientists tried to link an increase in human brain cancer between the late 1970s and mid 1980s to a higher use of aspartame, but further analysis exposed inconsistencies in their data. Long-term studies on laboratory rats have found no harmful effects from the consumption of aspartame. In September 2007, a panel of 10 American researchers conducted a review of more than 500 aspartame studies and concluded that it is safe. However, if you consume moderate or large amounts of artificial sweetener, I recommend you consider the studies and decide for yourself.

Sucralose: Commonly known as Splenda. Sucralose is a sugar molecule. To create Splenda, sucralose undergoes a number of chemical alterations, including the addition of a chlorine atom. Splenda has only been on the market since 1998, thus we lack long-term studies on its side effects. The studies that have been conducted so far have failed to prove that it is harmful. David L. Katz, MD, MPH, director of the Yale Griffin Prevention Research Center in New Haven, Connecticut, told the *Los Angeles Times*, "There is no direct evidence that Splenda causes cancer. It's just a theoretical concern." That said, I caution my clients to use any artificial sweetener, including Splenda, in moderation. And remember, a little goes a long way.

Stevia: Stevia is a shrub whose leaves have long been used by the people of South America and Asia to sweeten beverages. Stevia is native to Paraguay and was used for decades in Japan to sweeten teas, cakes, and other products after saccharin was banned there in the 1970s. As of this writing, stevia is not approved for use as a food additive in the United States or Europe, so it is currently sold as a dietary supplement in health food stores. The FDA has reviewed little research on the use of

Skinny Chick Chat

Hey Christine! I grew up having dessert after every meal (okay, maybe not breakfast, but definitely lunch and dinner) and often sweet snacks in between. When I try to diet and cut out sweets altogether, I give up after a week or so. Can I have my sweets and diet too?

SARAH H., CHICAGO

Sarah: Yes you can—in moderation, of course. Just try some of the recipes beginning on page 280. If you go out to eat and you crave dessert, split one with your dinner companions. The caveat is that these desserts should be eaten shortly after a small, balanced meal or eaten with a lean protein. I have separated the nutrition in each meal on my program so you can easily swap any carb and fat for a reasonable serving of your favorite dessert. Combining these tasty treats with a lean protein will help slow the speed of the sugar from these foods as its glucose molecules flow down the Blood Sugar Freeway. It is important to realize that one enormous dessert can throw off the stability of your blood sugar level for up to 3 days.

EAT WELL, CHRISTINE

stevia and found concerns that it may be related to cancer development. This has not been proved, and stevia has an excellent safety profile in Japan, where it has been used for more than 30 years in foods. In the early 1990s, the FDA concluded that "available toxicological information on stevia is inadequate to demonstrate its safety as a food additive." On the other hand, in 2006, the World Health Organization published a report stating that it found no major toxicity risks, but it said more data is needed on stevia's effect on hypertension and blood sugar levels. Stevia is approximately 200 times sweeter than sugar and virtually calorie free. If you choose to use it, use it in moderation.

Agave nectar: This is a wonderful natural sweetener and a great alternative to artificial sweeteners in my opinion. However, agave nectar is not calorie free; it yields 20 calories per teaspoon. Agave nectar is derived from the heart of a Mexican cactus, which contains a sweet-sticky juice. In the 1500s, when the Spaniards arrived in Mexico, they fermented the juice of the agave plant into what we know today as tequila. More recently, agave syrup has hit the health food stores as a fantastic alternative sweetener for health-conscious individuals. The great thing about agave nectar is that it is approximately 90 percent fructose, so it has a low glycemic level, which, as we know, is helpful when it comes to keeping blood sugar levels steady. This makes agave a natural healthy option for people with diabetes and all people who are concerned about their waistlines. I personally use about a tablespoon of this sweetener almost every day, both in my morning tea and in my yummy Greek yogurt parfait (see the recipe on page 122).

To wrap it all up, remember that Skinny Chicks don't eat salads. They eat real foods, and they do have desserts once in a while. They don't need a separate splurge day because they eat healthfully most of the time, and if they want dessert, they pair it up with a protein and eat it as part of a meal. If you build up that "poor me, I'm so deprived" diet mind-set and never allow yourself a splurge, you're bound for a major binge. So follow the Skinny Chicks' dessert guidelines and have a sweet life!

SKINNY CHICKS' DESSERT GUIDELINES

1. If you're going to have dessert, have it with your meal.

2. Eat a lean protein before your dessert.

3. Swap a starchy carbohydrate from your entrée for your dessert, omitting rice, potato, fruits, or breads.

4. Your dessert portion should be low in fat and less than 50 grams of carbohydrates.

5. Do not have a dessert more than twice a week if you truly want to lose weight.

6. To jump-start weight loss, hold off on dessert until you've reached your goal weight.

CHAPTER 16

The Diner's Dilemma

When I was growing up and living with my grandparents, they prepared every meal at home. We had breakfast and lunch together every single day (when I was in school, Grandma packed me a sandwich), and every night at 6:00 p.m. there was food on the table. Many households across the country were the same. When the family dinner was still part of our society, you rarely saw the Styrofoam and plastic containers full of take-out food that have become such a fixture in today's American kitchens. Cooking at home is almost a quaint notion for many people—sort of a nostalgic memory of a simpler time. Nutritionally speaking, that has been to our detriment. When you cook at home, there is no question that the food you eat is healthier and less fattening, not to mention less expensive, and it's nice to have something delicious filling the kitchen with great aromas. As they say, "when you cook, you're family." That is why I have created a multitude of quick and easy meal preparations that fit into my nutrition program nicely and, in most cases, can be prepared in less than 10 minutes.

But one thing you can be sure of is that unless you are living with your own parents or grandparents, many of your meals will be coming from food stands, delis, fast-food joints, and restaurants. It is an inescapable fact of modern American life that few of us have time to make many, much less most, of our meals at home. Therefore it is vitally important to have a plan for ordering the right food when eating out.

Restaurants want you to enjoy the taste of their food, and if that means a little more oil or butter, then that is what they will use. Even when you order healthy restaurant choices, you will consume more fat than you would if you prepared the same thing at home; if you choose a less healthy preparation, such as something deep-fried, who knows how much fat you are consuming? But the worst thing about eating out is that most people can't resist all the extras—a warm, soft brownie, a raspberry lemonade, a side of curly fries, a new coffee drink with whipped cream, the bread before the meal and the dessert afterward. People who eat out often end up consuming a lot of these calorie-laden add-ons, and it can make weight control impossible. Even if you eat only one or two of these extras per week, you may sabotage your weight loss—or, even worse, gain weight.

Meet Rachelle, Who Had the Belly Fat Blues

Rachelle, a 19-year-old UCLA student, came to see me to lose the extra belly fat she had gained during her freshman year. She was tall, pretty, and mostly slender, but her belly area was round and protruding. I reviewed her food journal and noticed that she and her friends ate at a restaurant every night. They would always start with bread and butter, maybe some chips and salsa, or sometimes potato skins or mozzarella cheese sticks. She didn't want to say no when her friends were eating, so she ate along with them. She told me that since she was eating all the extra stuff, she usually just ordered a salad for dinner (and we know how that works). When dessert time rolled around, they would split a dessert among them. All these little extras had the not surprising effect of saddling Rachelle with the dreaded freshman 15.

When I explained to Rachelle about blood sugar and the PC Combo, she said, "Wow, that's all I have to do? I'll try it." She took the info and ran with it. In 10 weeks, she lost 14 pounds and looked fantastic. She was overflowing with confidence and personality. Now, when she met up with friends for dinner, she no longer felt out of control, so she could easily say no to the mozzarella stick and nacho appetizers. When she'd order a substantial entrée, her friends would pepper her with questions about how she could

Skinny Chick 10-Week Transformation

NAME: JENNIFER K.

AGE: 37

TOTAL POUNDS LOST: 21

TOTAL INCHES LOST: 22

In my mind, I have been overweight all my life. As an adult, I'm finally realizing that the childhood image I've always held of myself (the fat girl) is untrue. Yes, I carried a few extra pounds, as a young girl rarely made good food choices, and spent more time reading or watching TV than recommended, but I didn't become truly obese until after high school.

One of my earliest memories is of a relative making me a breakfast different from my brother's because "it was time for me to lose some weight." I can remember being surprised and actually thinking, *When did it go from baby fat to just fat?* I was 7 or 8 years old. So I struggled.

After high school, I embarked on a low-fat diet. I counted fat grams and did lose inches and weight—but I gained it back. At 25 years old, after a major breakup, I finally did it right. I ate healthy meals prepared at home, exercised regularly, and enjoyed once-monthly "cheat weekends," where pizza and brownies were meals of choice. That lasted 5 months, but when I moved in with roommates, I reverted to the old habits. I was self-conscious about exercising where people could see me, and I ate what they cooked rather than rocking the boat.

Today, I make better choices more often, but for the most part, this has only stopped the weight gain rather than inducing weight loss. I am still rather inactive, and my old friends, books and TV, are never far away.

The best thing about the Skinny Chicks program is that my whole outlook on life has changed since I started. I am working to alter my relationship with food, and this plan has allowed me to really define and enjoy the healthy foods available to me. I certainly have noticed that my body is changing. Both my stomach and my rear end have become smaller. I have much more energy, which allows me to participate in many more things than I was previously doing. I believe I am making much better choices for myself, and I definitely plan to stick with this program for the long haul.

Since I started the program, I eat more often than I used to. I take supplements. I am aware of the best options for me, and I don't have to have a meal loaded with unhealthy carbs in order to enjoy what I'm eating. I now look forward to a meal that not only tastes good, but that also has nutritional value as well.

eat the meals she was eating and still lose weight. She had to tell them that her foods were actually a lot healthier than their salads. Ten weeks, a flat tummy, and 14 pounds later, her friends were convinced.

Your Best Bets Eating Out

Once you've gotten a handle on all those diet-busting extras, the next thing to do is figure out what in the world to order. Don't worry; no matter where you choose to dine, I guarantee you can find great healthy choices to keep you on your plan. I have designed meal plans that include favorite restaurants for more than 1,000 of my clients. While many people lament the fact that the exact same chain restaurants appear in every city in America, in this case it's a good thing, because it means my suggestions will work no matter where you live. Here are some helpful examples:

- **Food stands:** Many of our meals come from a cafeteria at work, a food court at the mall, or some other food stand–type location. What can you order from these places and stay on your food plan? I always look for a selection that contains a nice helping of chicken breast, turkey, or fish along with a healthy carb. Examples: chicken or fish soft tacos, deli turkey sandwiches, tomato-based pasta with chicken, chicken burritos (hold the sour cream and cheese), chicken teriyaki with rice, turkey burgers on a wheat roll, grilled chicken/salmon/ahi tuna sandwiches, and, in the mornings, egg white sandwiches (hold the cheese). If there is too much sauce, butter, mayonnaise, or cheese on your food, just scrape some of it off. Every little bit of these high-fat items makes a big difference. (You can use all the ketchup, mustard, and salsa you want.) The things to avoid are your standard fare: hot dogs, hamburgers, fries, nachos, shakes, cinnamon rolls, and ice cream. Watch out for those "garden burgers," which, surprisingly, are often loaded with fat. You are much better off going for a turkey burger without the cheese. Avoid any fried foods, cream sauces, and regular sodas.

- **Delis:** Delis are a great place to grab a healthy bite. Order a smoked turkey, chicken breast, or lean ham sandwich with no cheese and light mayo, then pile on the veggies to your heart's content. The things to avoid are tuna salad or chicken salad sandwiches, salami and processed meats, and regular cheese. Don't get tricked by the special veggie sandwiches with regular cheese: They are very high in fat.

- **Casual restaurants/diners/takeout:** Almost every neighborhood in America has an Italian, Mexican, and Asian eatery. If you're lucky, you also have Thai, Indian, and Greek spots, as well as a good old American diner or two. Then of course there are the inescapable chain restaurants. All of these provide us with many healthy food options for dining in or taking home. Again, I recommend looking for dishes that are based on chicken, turkey, or fish and sometimes lean steak (preferably filet mignon, if you can afford it). Here is a partial list of my favorites:

  - **Asian:** Chicken stir-fry or chicken teriyaki plus a side salad; hold the dressing and use rice vinegar
  - **Diner:** Roasted turkey breast with a baked potato, hold the mashed
  - **Greek:** Chicken skewers with rice; hold the hummus
  - **Grill:** Grilled fish with rice and veggies; hold the oil; use lemon and herbs for seasoning
  - **Indian:** Chicken tikka with rice and veggies; hold the masala cream sauce
  - **Italian:** Pasta with tomato sauce with chicken or shrimp, plus a side salad (use balsamic vinegar instead of dressing); hold the cheese and cream sauces
  - **Mexican:** Grilled chicken or shrimp fajitas or tacos; hold the guacamole, cheese, and sour cream
  - **Thai:** Garlic chicken with rice and steamed veggies

  This list could go on and on, but I think you get the idea. You'll find that healthy choices are available no matter what type of restaurant you frequent, if you are vigilant about holding the high-fat extras like cheese and sour cream.

Look for the dishes that are based on healthy lean proteins. What should you avoid? As we know, those specialty salads tend to be extremely high in calories and fat. Anything with a creamy sauce is going to be overloaded with fat (fettuccine Alfredo would be enemy number one). Anything involving cheese, sour cream, butter, or lots of oil (such as deep-fried foods) is definitely on the "best to avoid" list. Remember that cheese, sour cream, and butter are animal-based high-fat foods whose fat is mostly saturated. Many, many dishes combine multiple high-fat offenders—like deep-fried mozzarella sticks dipped in ranch dressing, or deep-fried fish tacos with sour cream. As you start to recognize the primary high-fat food sources, it becomes easier to find healthful choices in your own life.

- **Fine dining:** When dining in a full-service restaurant, my best advice is that you eat a small meal 2 hours before your reservation. Often you wind up sitting down an hour late for various reasons, and you don't want to be starving. Try not to eat the bread before dinner. This isn't always easy to do when you sit down to eat and you are so hungry that you're ready to gnaw on your own arm. But bread on an empty stomach causes a rapid rise in blood sugar. Better to order a chicken skewer or a crab or shrimp cocktail (something that is primarily protein) as an appetizer right away and have the waiter take the bread back where it came from.

When you do order your entrée, again stay away from the high-fat foods: cream sauces, cheesy dishes, fried foods, and oily or buttery dishes. Stay with tomato-based sauces and grilled meat cuts such as fish, chicken, and filet mignon.

For all of my specifics, refer to the meal plans found in Chapter 11, which include healthy choices from many favorite American restaurants. Additionally, I have created a "fast-food guide" at www.christineavanti.com for inquiring minds who want to know the best and worst fast-food eats. I recommend you check it out if you are not able to prepare your own meals on a regular basis. I'm not a fan of fast food, but I realize that in today's world, the reality is most people wind up eating at fast-food restaurants more often than anywhere else.

CHAPTER 17

Skinny Chicks' Helpful Tricks

Life isn't perfect. That's one of the things that makes "dieting" so hard. I'm asking you to make changes in your lifestyle: to eat every 4 hours, to combine carbs and proteins, to exercise five times a week. If you are able to do all those things all the time, more power to you. If you can't, all it means is that you're a human being. If you can't always follow the plan perfectly every time, don't worry; it's not the end of the world. If perfection were the only goal, few people would make it past the second day. Don't cave in and have a huge binge; just get right back on your plan.

Fortunately, there are lots of options for keeping your weight loss going even when life throws you a curveball. This chapter will help you cope when that happens.

Timing Is Everything

What if you can't eat on the 4-hour mark? What if you're invited to a fabulous party where everyone will be eating all kinds of food for 5 straight hours? What if you were stuck at work and couldn't eat for 8 hours—and then had three doughnuts? What if it is a holiday or somebody's birthday? What if your life is not regimented with military precision?

Most of us do not run our lives with military precision, and we really wouldn't want to. With some foresight and planning, though, you can still fit in the meals you need to keep your brain supplied with glucose and thus keep your body lean and mean. Let's say your plan calls for you to eat at 8:00 a.m., 12:00 p.m., and 4:00 p.m., but you are invited to a dinner party at 6:00 p.m. Rather than starve yourself until 6:00 (and more than likely overeat at dinner), just cut your 4:00 p.m. meal in half, then go have dinner at 6:00 p.m. (I recommend that you have a half-meal here, unless you are tremendously hungry; in that case, have a full meal and wait 4 hours until your next meal if you are still awake at that time.) As long as you eat the proper balance of nutrients at every meal, you will be fine. You may actually have as many as six small meals in a given day. As long as you keep them balanced and modestly portioned, you'll be sticking to your plan. In fact, this is very similar to the way professional athletes and celebrities eat.

Let's look at some specific situations and strategies for coping with them.

The Mega-Binge Disaster: Social Obligations

What if you find yourself at a huge dinner party where you are served seven courses? Many of my socially active clients have this dilemma. In 2004, I began working with a client by the name of Kallissa. Kallissa started the Skinny Chicks program at 28 percent body fat and ended at 19 percent, and she has been able to maintain her results for more than 3 years despite her very busy work and social schedule. Here is Kallissa's story.

Kallissa was an avid exerciser and healthful eater for many years, but her career as an executive producer of three hit shows on MTV made it nearly impossible for her to stick to her goals. Kallissa had a staff of more than 150 people, and to reward their hard work, Kallissa liked to throw fun events for holidays and premieres, and wrap parties. This added up to two or three major parties each month, and that did not include the other social commitments that come with the territory of being a Hollywood producer. With a schedule like Kallissa's, you'd think it would be almost impossible to adhere to my Skinny Chicks nutrition plan. Kallissa asked me for tips on how to navigate her way through these events so that she could continue on the plan in a way that would not be obvious to onlookers.

Here are some of the tips I gave her:

- **Never go to an event on an empty stomach.** Kallissa often ate reduced-fat string cheese and a small piece of fruit in the car on her way to an event or hot spot.

- **Nurse one drink all night** (see page 289 for low-calorie beverages). When Kallissa arrived at a function, she would order a glass of champagne (approximately 5 ounces) and sip on this 100-calorie beverage for an hour or even 2 hours, during which time her colleagues might have had three or four drinks.

- **Order food before you start drinking.** If you're going to a bar or restaurant where food is served, eat first, *then* drink. If you start with alcohol, you're more likely to give in to temptation and have something outside your plan. I advised Kallissa to order a lean protein prepared with very little oil and some high-fiber carbohydrates such as brown rice or steamed veggies. Kallissa's favorite "bar" meal was shrimp cocktail, one or two bites of another appetizer if one was ordered by someone in her party, and one glass of champagne.

- **Don't punish yourself for slipping up.** I usually tell my clients to try to avoid challenging social situations for the first 10 weeks of the Skinny Chicks program, but I know that's not always possible. If you do go out and you do slip up, don't starve yourself the next day. Simply go right back to your plan. Weight loss, like life, doesn't go in a straight line; there are ups and downs. If you go right back to your plan, your weight will continue to drop.

Anticipate Starvation Solutions

What if you are stuck on the road or at work and can't take a break to eat? What if you are in an important meeting and eating is out of the question?

These are the toughest situations and the ones I find the toughest to deal with. My office gets so busy at times that my scheduled meal breaks get absorbed if a client shows up late, or an appointment goes past its allotted 30 minutes. When I miss an appointed meal time by an hour, two, or even more, I start to feel a little loopy. At times like these, making good food choices is almost impossible. Often, I am so short on time that I only have 5 minutes to run down and grab something from the Starbucks coffee bar in my building. By that time, I'm starving and feel tempted to order the maple scone and a double mocha. I have to remind myself to take a deep breath and calm down. I tell myself, "Look. You're hungry and your blood sugar is low. Just stick with the plan and you'll be fine." Then I order a turkey sandwich and fruit cup . . . and I feel more energized than if I had had the double mocha and scone.

The key is to *anticipate* these situations and eat before they happen. Keep a high-fiber protein bar in your purse, briefcase, or car. I don't recommend these as meal replacements, and they may contain additives I'd rather avoid, but in a pinch they are far better than a pastry or greasy fast food. If you're trapped in a meeting, use the bathroom breaks to eat a quick bite and keep your blood sugar on an even keel. That's the best way to stay sharp—and on your plan.

Be Efficient

One great strategy to help avoid missing meals is to cook or buy more than one meal at a time. Your life is busy; why should you spend more time than you have to shopping, preparing, and cleaning up? If you are going to cook, make enough for two or three meals so you can have leftovers. The same goes for ordering takeout or eating out. If you are getting lunch to go, buy enough so you can eat some now and some for your late afternoon meal. If you eat dinner in a restaurant, plan to take some home for tomorrow night's dinner. This way, you are unlikely to overeat (restaurant portions can be *huge!*), and you'll already have one of tomorrow's meals ready to go. This is also a great help when you get hungry and you want something to eat *right now*. If you have leftovers readily available, you're less likely to veer off your plan.

Meet Dr. John, the Coke Fiend

One of my clients, John, was an ophthalmologist. He was in his sixties and appeared to be in decent shape; he was tall and thin. He had been referred to me by his own doctor after an annual checkup. Despite his mostly healthy appearance, his blood work showed that he was prediabetic, so his doctor recommended that I review his diet.

I reviewed his food journal and discovered that he ate nothing all day long, then had a large dinner at night. The only thing that kept him going during the day was quaffing a Coke whenever he had a break. With each Coke, John's body would receive a massive infusion of sugar.

John said, "I don't have time to eat. I see patients all day long. In between patients, I drink Coca-Cola and that's all the time I've got. Besides that, I love drinking Coke, so don't tell me to quit."

I told him he had to start eating breakfast every day and have his secretaries schedule time between patients for lunch and one midafternoon meal. Now, bear in mind, this is a successful medical professional who was not overweight. When I laid out his meal plans and showed him that they did not include Cokes, he was impatient and very annoyed.

"Aww c'mon, there's got to be something else. Can't you give me a supplement or some kind of drink? You can't be serious. How can I eat real food all day long? Why should I pay you to tell me to give up my Cokes? I am *not* giving up my Cokes, and I also like having a dessert at night." The concept of eating real food during the day seemed inconvenient and as foreign to John as reading Chinese. Cokes, on the other hand, were easy and readily available.

At this point, I got dead serious with John. "Do you have a family?" I asked.

"Yes."

"Do you have kids?"

"Yes."

"Do you have grandkids?"

"Yes."

"Do you want to see them grow up?"

"Well, of course!"

"Then you are going to have to start eating real food and stabilizing your blood sugar or you won't. You are prediabetic and, being a doctor, you should know what happens to diabetic people who do not eat properly. They can end up on dialysis, go blind, lose extremities to amputation, and eventually die from their condition." For some reason it hadn't occurred to John that his all-soda diet was literally ushering him to an early grave. Reluctantly, he decided to try my plan. He started eating breakfast and quick but balanced meals twice a day between patients. Although weight loss was not his goal, he ended up losing 10 pounds and reducing his body fat by 3 percent by the 10th week of my program.

More importantly, 2 months later, a blood test showed that John was no longer prediabetic. He was in much brighter spirits and had more energy. He smiled as he told me that his secretaries said he had been a much nicer person over the past 2 months. The unstable blood sugar levels had been causing his moods to go haywire. John's 30-year habit had seemed to work for him, but inside, his body was calling out for a change. The happy result? John has put his life back on a healthy track, he has avoided diabetes, and he has made life better for all the people around him.

PART V

SKINNY CHICKS

GET IN

THE KITCHEN

Recipes

In this section, you'll find recipes for all the dishes mentioned in the meal plans on pages 122 through 165, plus extra breakfast, lunch, dinner, and dessert recipes for planning your own menus.

By now I hope you have realized that it's not just how *much* you eat but what you eat that matters. Sure, you could satisfy your body's need for fuel—and probably come up with perfectly adequate PC combos—by defrosting a frozen entrée for every meal. But choosing top-quality ingredients and preparing them with care will result in meals that satisfy so much more than just your basic physiological needs.

As a child, I often spent weekends with my grandparents on their ranch. In the morning, I was up early to pick fruits and vegetables with Grandpa Luigi for the big Sunday afternoon feast—a tradition we never missed. My entire family—grandparents, aunts, uncles, cousins, my mom, my two sisters, and me—gathered around the table to eat a wonderful meal cooked with love by my grandmother. As we walked through the ranch, Grandpa taught me about growing and caring for the fruits, vegetables, and herbs—and about life.

Anybody who has ever eaten fresh farm-grown produce knows how much better it tastes than commercially farmed products. From the fresh salad to the homemade pasta to the ranch-raised meat to the homemade wine, the whole meal was balanced, homegrown, and homemade, with plenty of variety.

Long before fad dieting ever started, Grandma and Grandpa were eating healthy, natural, nutritious meals from the earth that included protein, carbohydrates, and fats. Sometimes in my research I can hear Grandpa Luigi saying, "Chris, a gooda meal is like a gooda lifa—needs a gooda balance."

When Grandpa Luigi passed away, his strength helped me through the tough times before I finally found my calling as a nutritionist. Today,

I think of him with every meal I make. Most importantly, I feel empowered by something Grandpa Luigi knew all along—that food is meant to be a joyful part of life that brings people together. Slowly and surely, as the Skinny Chicks program came together, the depressed, hopeless feelings of futility so familiar to dieters were replaced by feelings of health and confidence, as the way I eat was changed forever.

These are the recipes that I've shared with my clients and that I prepare nightly for myself and my husband. Paired with the grab-and-go suggestions you'll find in the meal plans, they keep us satisfied, well nourished, and happy at the table. I hope you will enjoy these recipes and be inspired to adapt some of your favorite recipes to PC combos, too!

Christine's High-Protein Pumpkin Ginger Pancakes

Nutrition facts per serving: 376 calories, 21 grams protein,
53 grams carbohydrates, 10 grams fat SERVES 4 (2 PANCAKES PER SERVING)

- -

1 cup whole grain flour

2 tablespoons brown sugar

1 teaspoon baking powder

½ teaspoon baking soda

½ teaspoon cinnamon

½ teaspoon ginger

¼ teaspoon salt

1 cup light vanilla soy milk

2 scoops protein powder
(any brand that yields
20 grams protein per scoop)

1 5-ounce container 0% Greek
vanilla bean yogurt

¾ cup canned pumpkin

2 extra-large egg whites

2 tablespoons butter,
slightly melted

2 slices crystallized ginger,
quarter-shaped, diced

2 tablespoons cold butter

Nonstick cooking spray

4 tablespoons maple syrup

In a large mixing bowl, combine the first 7 ingredients and set aside.

In a blender, combine the soy milk and protein powder and blend for
30 seconds, then pour into a medium bowl. To the protein mixture, add the
yogurt, pumpkin, egg whites, and butter and mix well.

Add the liquid mixture to the dry ingredients and stir just until moist.
Do not overmix the pancake batter.

Warm a griddle or large skillet over medium-low heat. Meanwhile, add the
ginger to the butter, mix well, and set aside.

Spray the heated griddle or skillet with cooking spray. Ladle the pancake
batter onto the griddle, using ¼ cup of batter for each pancake. Let each
pancake cook for 2 to 3 minutes per side. Spread lightly with ginger butter
and ½ tablespoon of syrup per cake.

PROTEIN POWERED	CARBOHYDRATE CONCENTRATED	FAT FRIENDLY	FREE FOODS
Protein powder, egg whites, fat-free Greek yogurt	Whole grain flour, sugar, soy milk, pumpkin, crystallized ginger, maple syrup	Butter, cooking spray	Baking powder, baking soda, cinnamon, ginger

Artichoke Frittata

Nutrition facts per serving: 351 calories, 25 grams protein, 43 grams carbohydrates, 9 grams fat SERVES 1

1 teaspoon extra virgin olive oil
½ cup liquid egg whites
½ cup fat-free milk
1 pinch each of salt and ground black pepper
1 tablespoon whole wheat flour
2 tablespoons grated reduced-fat Parmesan cheese
¼ cup artichoke hearts in water, drained and chopped
1 whole grain English muffin, toasted

Preheat the oven to 350°F. Brush a mini loaf pan with the oil and set aside.

In a medium bowl, whisk together the egg whites, milk, and salt and pepper. Then whisk in the flour and cheese and fold in the artichokes.

Pour the egg mixture into the prepared loaf pan.

Bake for 10 minutes.

Cover with foil and bake another 5 to 10 minutes. The frittata is done when a toothpick comes out clean.

Serve with the English muffin.

PROTEIN POWERED	CARBOHYDRATE CONCENTRATED	FAT FRIENDLY	FREE FOODS
Egg whites, fat-free milk, Parmesan cheese	Artichoke hearts, whole grain English muffin	Extra virgin olive oil	Salt and ground black pepper

Nutrition facts calculated by Menu Magic Personal Chef Software, Version 2.6, 2008, Kreotek, LLC, Rio Rancho, New Mexico.

CHRISTINE'S NUTRITION NUGGETS Artichokes are a fantastic source of vitamin C (good for skin and immunity), folate (important for cell division during pregnancy), and potassium (good for cellular fluid balance).

Blueberry Blintzes

Nutrition facts per serving: 391 calories, 28 grams protein,
56 grams carbohydrates, 6 grams fat SERVES 4 (3 BLINTZES PER SERVING)

2 cups low-fat cottage cheese

8 ounces fat-free cream cheese

$\frac{1}{2}$ cup liquid egg whites

$\frac{1}{3}$ cup blueberry preserves

1 tablespoon lemon juice

Nonstick cooking spray

12 store-bought crepe shells

1 cup fresh blueberries

Preheat the oven to 350°F.

Mix the first 5 ingredients together in a bowl until well combined.

Spray a large baking pan with cooking spray.

Place 2 crepe shells flat onto the baking pan, and put one-twelfth of the cheese mixture into the center of each crepe.

Shape the crepe shell into a rectangle by loosely folding in the short ends of the crepe shell first, and then each of the sides.

Repeat for the remaining crepes.

Bake for 12 to 15 minutes, or until golden brown.

Top with the fresh blueberries.

PROTEIN POWERED	CARBOHYDRATE CONCENTRATED	FAT FRIENDLY	FREE FOODS
Cottage cheese, cream cheese, egg whites	Blueberry preserves, crepes, blueberries	Cooking spray	Lemon juice

Nutrition facts calculated by Menu Magic Personal Chef Software, Version 2.6, 2008, Kreotek, LLC, Rio Rancho, New Mexico.

CHRISTINE'S NUTRITION NUGGETS Blueberries are one of the highest antioxidant-loaded fruits, and they contain pectin, a good fiber that binds to toxins. They also contain a compound, epicatechin, similar to that found in cranberries, that helps prevent urinary tract infections.

Breakfast Bagel Sandwich

Nutrition facts per serving: 369 calories, 27 grams protein, 44 grams carbohydrates, 9 grams fat SERVES 1

1 oat bran bagel

Nonstick cooking spray

1 slice extra-lean turkey bacon

1 teaspoon omega-3 light spread

½ cup liquid egg whites

1 pinch each of salt and ground black pepper

2 tablespoons reduced-fat cream cheese

1 small tomato, sliced

Toast the bagel and set aside.

Coat a nonstick pan with cooking spray and cook the turkey bacon over medium-low heat.

When the bacon is cooked, remove it from the pan and set aside. Add the omega-3 spread to the pan.

Pour in the egg whites and sprinkle with the salt and pepper. While the egg is setting, chop the bacon.

When most of the egg is set, use a spatula to loosen the egg from the pan, allowing any uncooked egg to run off into the pan.

Sprinkle the chopped bacon onto the egg while it's still wet. Then fold in the sides of the egg to make a square. Flip the egg square to finish cooking.

Spread the cream cheese onto the bagel.

When the egg is firm, place it on the bagel, add the tomato, and serve.

PROTEIN POWERED	CARBOHYDRATE CONCENTRATED	FAT FRIENDLY	FREE FOODS
Turkey bacon, egg whites, cream cheese	Bagel	Cooking spray, omega-3 spread	Tomato

Nutrition facts calculated by Menu Magic Personal Chef Software, Version 2.6, 2008, Kreotek, LLC, Rio Rancho, New Mexico.

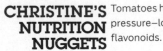 **CHRISTINE'S NUTRITION NUGGETS** Tomatoes have plenty of immune-boosting vitamin C, blood pressure–lowering potassium, and potential cancer-fighting flavonoids.

Canadian Bacon Breakfast Quesadilla

Nutrition facts per serving: 383 calories, 30 grams protein,
43 grams carbohydrates, 10 grams fat SERVES 2

2 large whole wheat tortillas

1½ teaspoons extra virgin olive oil

½ cup shredded fat-free Cheddar cheese

2 slices lean Canadian bacon, chopped

⅓ cup canned black beans, rinsed and drained

¼ cup chopped red bell pepper

¼ cup chopped red onion

Preheat the oven to 350°F.

Brush one side of each tortilla with the oil and place oil side down on a baking sheet.

Mix the remaining ingredients together in a bowl.

Divide the mixture into two. Spread each onto half of a tortilla. Fold the open side of each tortilla over onto the mix, forming a half-moon shape.

Bake for approximately 10 minutes, or until the tortillas are slightly crispy and the cheese has melted.

PROTEIN POWERED	CARBOHYDRATE CONCENTRATED	FAT FRIENDLY	FREE FOODS
Cheddar cheese, Canadian bacon	Whole wheat tortillas, black beans	Extra virgin olive oil	Red bell pepper, red onion

Nutrition facts calculated by Menu Magic Personal Chef Software, Version 2.6, 2008, Kreotek, LLC, Rio Rancho, New Mexico.

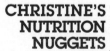

CHRISTINE'S NUTRITION NUGGETS Canadian bacon has 1.5 grams of fat per ounce, which is far lower in fat than regular bacon at 11 grams of fat per ounce. If you don't like Canadian bacon, you can use low-sodium turkey deli slices, which are fat free!

Cinnamon Raisin Oatmeal Muffins

Nutrition facts per serving: 394 calories, 25 grams protein,
54 grams carbohydrates, 9 grams fat SERVES 4 (3 MUFFINS PER SERVING)
• •

Nonstick cooking spray

1⅓ cups liquid egg whites

1⅓ cups low-fat cottage cheese

¼ cup omega-3 light spread

1⅓ cups oats

¾ cup raisins, chopped

3 tablespoons cinnamon

2 teaspoons stevia (see page 215)

3 tablespoons vanilla-flavored egg white protein powder

Preheat the oven to 350°F.

Spray a 12-cup muffin pan with cooking spray.

In a large bowl, mix the egg whites, cottage cheese, and omega-3 spread until thoroughly combined.

Add the oats and mix well. Stir in the remaining ingredients.

Divide the batter among the prepared muffin cups.

Bake for 25 to 30 minutes. The muffins are done when a toothpick inserted into the center of a muffin comes out clean.

PROTEIN POWERED	CARBOHYDRATE CONCENTRATED	FAT FRIENDLY	FREE FOODS
Egg whites, cottage cheese, protein powder	Oats, raisins	Cooking spray, omega-3 spread	Cinnamon, stevia

Nutrition facts calculated by Menu Magic Personal Chef Software, Version 2.6, 2008, Kreotek, LLC, Rio Rancho, New Mexico.

Denver Omelet
with Breakfast Potatoes

Nutrition facts per serving: 365 calories, 26 grams protein,
47 grams carbohydrates, 8 grams fat SERVES 1

1 medium russet potato, cubed

⅓ cup chopped onion, divided

1 teaspoon extra virgin olive oil

1 pinch each of salt and ground black pepper

½ cup liquid egg whites

¼ cup fat-free milk

Nonstick cooking spray

2 slices lean Canadian bacon, chopped

1 tablespoon chopped green bell pepper

Preheat the oven to 375ºF. On a sheet pan, toss the potato and ¼ cup of the onion in the oil. Season with the salt and black pepper. Spread out into an even layer. Bake approximately 20 minutes, or until the potato is brown and crispy.

In a small bowl, whisk the egg whites and milk together.

Spray a nonstick pan with cooking spray and warm over medium heat. Pour the egg mixture into the pan and let set 1 to 2 minutes. Lift the sides of the omelet to let the uncooked egg run off.

Add the Canadian bacon, bell pepper, and remaining onion to half of the omelet, and fold in half. When the bottom is slightly brown, flip the omelet and let cook another 1 to 2 minutes.

Serve with the potatoes.

PROTEIN POWERED	CARBOHYDRATE CONCENTRATED	FAT FRIENDLY	FREE FOODS
Egg whites, fat-free milk, Canadian bacon	Potato	Extra virgin olive oil, cooking spray	Onion, green bell pepper

Nutrition facts calculated by Menu Magic Personal Chef Software, Version 2.6, 2008, Kreotek, LLC, Rio Rancho, New Mexico.

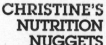

CHRISTINE'S NUTRITION NUGGETS Egg whites are an excellent source of protein, amino acids, zinc, and B vitamins.

Protein-Powered Vanilla French Toast

Nutrition facts per serving: 360 calories, 25 grams protein, 47 grams carbohydrates, 7 grams fat SERVES 4

. . . .

1 1/3 cups liquid egg whites

1/2 cup vanilla-flavored egg white protein powder, Jay Robb's brand (found at Whole Foods stores)

1 tablespoon vanilla extract

1/4 cup omega-3 light spread

8 large slices whole wheat bread

1 cup fresh strawberries

1/2 cup fat-free whipped topping

In a medium bowl, whisk together the first 3 ingredients and set aside.

Melt the omega-3 spread as needed in a large nonstick pan over medium heat.

Dip the bread into the egg mixture, coating both sides of each slice well.

Cook the bread approximately 2 minutes on each side, or until golden.

Top with the strawberries and whipped topping.

PROTEIN POWERED	CARBOHYDRATE CONCENTRATED	FAT FRIENDLY	FREE FOODS
Egg whites, protein powder	Whole wheat bread, strawberries	Omega-3 spread	Vanilla extract, fat-free whipped topping

Nutrition facts calculated by Menu Magic Personal Chef Software, Version 2.6, 2008, Kreotek, LLC, Rio Rancho, New Mexico.

CHRISTINE'S NUTRITION NUGGETS Omega-3 spread is similar to soft margarines, but it is trans fat free and a great source of heart-healthy essential fatty acids.

Huevos and Potatoes Rancheros

Nutrition facts per serving: 343 calories, 25 grams protein, 44 grams carbohydrates, 7 grams fat SERVES 1

. . . .

1 medium russet potato

1 teaspoon extra virgin olive oil

1 pinch each of salt and ground black pepper

Nonstick cooking spray

²/₃ cup liquid egg whites

¹/₃ cup enchilada sauce

2 tablespoons shredded fat-free Cheddar cheese

2 tablespoons chopped scallions

1 teaspoon chopped fresh cilantro

Preheat the oven to 375°F. Slice the potato into ¼" rounds. Place on a baking sheet and toss with the oil and salt and pepper. Spread out in an even layer.

Bake for 15 minutes. A fork should easily go through the potato slices when done.

Coat a nonstick pan with cooking spray and place over medium heat. Add the egg whites and cook, stirring as needed to scramble. Spread the eggs over the potato. Top with the enchilada sauce. Sprinkle with the cheese, scallions, and cilantro.

PROTEIN POWERED	CARBOHYDRATE CONCENTRATED	FAT FRIENDLY	FREE FOODS
Egg whites, Cheddar cheese	Potato, enchilada sauce	Extra virgin olive oil, cooking spray	Scallions, cilantro

Nutrition facts calculated by Menu Magic Personal Chef Software, Version 2.6, 2008, Kreotek, LLC, Rio Rancho, New Mexico.

CHRISTINE'S NUTRITION NUGGETS Scallions not only add great flavor to this meal, but they are also part of the allyl sulfur compound family. One benefit of this compound family is that they (scallions) can help to improve cells' sensitivity to insulin and leptin (the satiety hormone).

Maple Walnut Ricotta Bake

Nutrition facts per serving: 402 calories, 26 grams protein,
58 grams carbohydrates, 7 grams fat SERVES 4

Nonstick cooking spray

1 cup fat-free ricotta cheese

2 cups liquid egg whites

1 tablespoon almond extract

1 cup fat-free milk

¾ cup light maple syrup

2 cups oat flour

1½ tablespoons chopped walnuts

Preheat the oven to 350ºF.

Spray an 11" × 7" baking dish with cooking spray.

In a large bowl, mix together the cheese, egg whites, almond extract, milk, and syrup.

Slowly stir in the flour until thoroughly combined.

Pour into the prepared baking dish and sprinkle the walnuts evenly on top.

Bake for 25 to 35 minutes. Test doneness by sticking a toothpick into the center. The bake is done when the toothpick comes out clean.

PROTEIN POWERED	CARBOHYDRATE CONCENTRATED	FAT FRIENDLY	FREE FOODS
Ricotta cheese, egg whites, fat-free milk	Maple syrup, oat flour	Cooking spray, ricotta cheese	Almond extract

Nutrition facts calculated by Menu Magic Personal Chef Software, Version 2.6, 2008, Kreotek, LLC, Rio Rancho, New Mexico.

CHRISTINE'S NUTRITION NUGGETS Oat flour is higher in fiber and nutrients than white flour, and it adds a nice texture.

Stuffed Breakfast Potato

Nutrition facts per serving: 370 calories, 25 grams protein, 44 grams carbohydrates, 8 grams fat SERVES 1

1 medium russet potato
2 strips extra-lean turkey bacon
$\frac{1}{2}$ cup liquid egg whites
1 pinch each of salt and ground black pepper
2 tablespoons Mexican cheese blend, 2% fat, divided
1 tablespoon chopped scallion, divided
$\frac{1}{4}$ cup fresh salsa, divided
1 tablespoon omega-3 light spread

Preheat the oven to 375ºF.

Poke the potato with a fork in several places. Microwave on high at 2-minute intervals, flipping and rotating the potato until soft, approximately 6 minutes total.

Meanwhile, cook the turkey bacon according to package directions, then chop. Set aside.

When the potato is ready, cut it in half and scoop out the center, leaving about $\frac{1}{2}$" of potato in the skin.

Mix the scooped-out potato with the bacon, egg whites, salt and pepper, and three-quarters each of the cheese, scallion, and salsa.

Melt the omega-3 spread in a nonstick pan over medium heat and cook the potato-egg mixture until the egg is still slightly moist.

Spoon the mixture into the potato skin and top with the remaining cheese, scallion, and salsa.

Bake for approximately 5 minutes, or until the cheese is melted and the potato is hot.

PROTEIN POWERED	CARBOHYDRATE CONCENTRATED	FAT FRIENDLY	FREE FOODS
Turkey bacon, egg whites, Mexican cheese	Potato	Omega-3 spread	Scallion, salsa

Nutrition facts calculated by Menu Magic Personal Chef Software, Version 2.6, 2008, Kreotek, LLC, Rio Rancho, New Mexico.

Southwest Scramble
with Corn Tortillas

Nutrition facts per serving: 382 calories, 25 grams protein,
50 grams carbohydrates, 9 grams fat SERVES 1

. . . .

½ cup liquid egg whites

¼ cup fat-free milk

1 pinch each of salt and ground black pepper

2 tablespoons canned diced green chile peppers

2 tablespoons chopped scallions

2 tablespoons corn

2 teaspoons omega-3 light spread

2 tablespoons Mexican cheese blend, 2% fat

3 corn tortillas

Salsa (optional)

In a small bowl, whisk together the egg whites, milk, and salt and black pepper. Stir in the chile peppers, scallions, and corn.

Melt the omega-3 spread in a nonstick pan over medium heat.

Pour the egg mixture into the pan and cook until the egg is still a little runny.

Add the cheese and cook until the cheese is melted and the egg is firm.

Wrap the tortillas in paper towels and microwave for 20 seconds.

Serve the eggs in the tortillas as tacos, or on the side if preferred.

PROTEIN POWERED	CARBOHYDRATE CONCENTRATED	FAT FRIENDLY	FREE FOODS
Egg whites, fat-free milk, Mexican cheese	Corn, corn tortillas	Omega-3 spread	Green chile peppers, scallions, salsa if you wish

Nutrition facts calculated by Menu Magic Personal Chef Software, Version 2.6, 2008, Kreotek, LLC, Rio Rancho, New Mexico.

CHRISTINE'S NUTRITION NUGGETS Eggs help to build white blood cells and antibodies that help fight illness and disease.

Berry Good Stuffed French Toast

Nutrition facts per serving: 390 calories, 23 grams protein,
53 grams carbohydrates, 8 grams fat SERVES 1

· ·

2 tablespoons low-sugar raspberry preserves

1 tablespoon fresh red raspberries

2 tablespoons light cream cheese

2 large slices whole wheat bread

½ cup liquid egg whites

Nonstick cooking spray

2 tablespoons fat-free whipped topping

1 mint leaf

In a small bowl, mix the preserves, raspberries, and cream cheese together until smooth.

Spread the mixture onto one side of one slice of bread and cover with the other slice to make a sandwich.

Pour the egg whites into a bowl. Dip and soak both sides of the sandwich in the eggs.

Coat a nonstick pan with cooking spray and warm over medium heat.

Cook the sandwich on each side for approximately 2 to 3 minutes, or until the egg is cooked and the sandwich is golden brown.

Garnish with the whipped topping and mint leaf.

PROTEIN POWERED	CARBOHYDRATE CONCENTRATED	FAT FRIENDLY	FREE FOODS
Light cream cheese, egg whites	Raspberry preserves, fresh raspberries, whole wheat bread	Cooking spray	Fat-free whipped topping, mint leaf

Nutrition facts calculated by Menu Magic Personal Chef Software, Version 2.6, 2008, Kreotek, LLC, Rio Rancho, New Mexico.

Zucchini and Mozzarella Strata

Nutrition facts per serving: 371 calories, 25 grams protein,
45 grams carbohydrates, 10 grams fat SERVES 4

• •

2 cups liquid egg whites

1 cup fat-free milk

2 medium zucchini, shredded

¼ cup chopped onion

½ cup shredded fat-free mozzarella cheese

1 teaspoon dried parsley

½ teaspoon salt

8 slices whole wheat bread

1½ tablespoons extra virgin olive oil

In a large bowl, whisk together the egg whites and milk. Stir in the zucchini, onion, cheese, parsley, and salt.

Break apart the bread into chunks and add to the egg mixture. Let soak at least 1 hour (can also soak overnight).

Preheat the oven to 350°F. Brush an 11" × 7" casserole dish with the oil.

Pour the strata mixture into the prepared dish and bake for 1 hour, or until a toothpick inserted in the center comes out clean.

PROTEIN POWERED	CARBOHYDRATE CONCENTRATED	FAT FRIENDLY	FREE FOODS
Egg whites, fat-free milk, fat-free mozzarella cheese	Whole wheat bread	Extra virgin olive oil	Zucchini, parsley

Nutrition facts calculated by Menu Magic Personal Chef Software, Version 2.6, 2008, Kreotek, LLC, Rio Rancho, New Mexico.

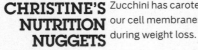 **CHRISTINE'S NUTRITION NUGGETS** Zucchini has carotenoids, which are known to protect our cell membranes from toxins that may be released during weight loss.

Asian Chicken Salad

Nutrition facts per serving: 335 calories, 28 grams protein,
42 grams carbohydrates, 8 grams fat SERVES 2

· ·

SALAD

2 medium chicken breasts,
grilled and diced

1 pound romaine lettuce,
inner leaves

2 ounces sugar snap peas

½ cup red bell pepper rings

1 cup shredded cabbage

1 tablespoon chopped cilantro

2 tablespoons Christine's Asian
Fusion Dressing

1 cup steamed brown rice

CHRISTINE'S ASIAN FUSION DRESSING

2 teaspoons sesame oil

1 teaspoon sesame seeds, toasted

¼ teaspoon brown sugar

1 tablespoon rice vinegar

1 tablespoon soy sauce

1 teaspoon fresh lime juice

1 teaspoon water

TO MAKE THE SALAD:

Combine the first 6 ingredients in a large bowl and serve with the Asian
dressing and rice on the side.

TO MAKE THE DRESSING:

Combine all of the ingredients in a small bowl and whisk for 30 seconds.

PROTEIN POWERED	CARBOHYDRATE CONCENTRATED	FAT FRIENDLY	FREE FOODS
Chicken breast	Sugar snap peas, brown rice	Asian fusion dressing	Romaine, red bell pepper, cabbage, cilantro

CHRISTINE'S NUTRITION NUGGETS Skinny chicks don't eat fattening salads, but they sure can enjoy a crisp and bountiful salad, loaded with healthy vegetables and a low-cal dressing. Just don't forget to have it with a healthy carb so that your blood sugar doesn't stay low, causing you to crave sugar a few hours later.

Thai Chicken Lettuce Cups

Nutrition facts per serving: 393 calories, 28 grams protein,
49 grams carbohydrates, 9 grams fat SERVES 4

- -

$\frac{1}{4}$ cup lime juice

$\frac{1}{2}$ cup light coconut milk

2 tablespoons reduced-fat creamy peanut butter

1 teaspoon crushed red-pepper flakes

10 ounces cooked boneless, skinless chicken breasts, chopped

2 cups cooked brown rice

12 butter lettuce or romaine leaves

1 cup shredded carrot

1 cup sliced cucumber

$1\frac{1}{3}$ cups mandarin oranges

$\frac{1}{4}$ cup chopped scallions

2 tablespoons chopped fresh cilantro

In a large bowl, mix the first 4 ingredients together until smooth.

Stir in the chicken and rice until well coated.

Divide the mixture into 12 piles and fill the lettuce leaves.

Add the remaining ingredients evenly on top of the lettuce cups.

PROTEIN POWERED	CARBOHYDRATE CONCENTRATED	FAT FRIENDLY	FREE FOODS
Chicken breast	Brown rice, carrot, mandarin oranges	Coconut milk, peanut butter	Lime juice, red-pepper flakes, romaine, cucumber, scallions, cilantro

Nutrition facts calculated by Menu Magic Personal Chef Software, Version 2.6, 2008, Kreotek, LLC, Rio Rancho, New Mexico.

CHRISTINE'S NUTRITION NUGGETS Mandarin oranges and carrots have high amounts of vitamin C, which has been shown in research studies to prevent stress-related weight gain, particularly in the belly.

Guiltless Turkey Nachos

Nutrition facts per serving: 381 calories, 28 grams protein,
45 grams carbohydrates, 10 grams fat SERVES 4
. . . .

3 large whole wheat tortillas

2 cups canned pinto beans, rinsed
and drained

Nonstick cooking spray

10 ounces lean ground turkey

2 teaspoons taco seasoning

1/2 cup crushed tomatoes

1/3 cup Mexican shredded cheese
blend, 2% fat

1/4 cup diced canned jalapeño
chile peppers

1/4 cup chopped scallions

2 tablespoons chopped fresh
cilantro

Preheat the oven to 375ºF.

Cut each tortilla into 16 chip-size pieces. Spread the pieces out on a baking
sheet and cook for 10 minutes or until crisp.

Transfer the chips to an ovenproof serving dish and spread the beans evenly
on top.

In a skillet coated with cooking spray, cook the turkey with the taco
seasoning over medium-high heat.

When the turkey is just slightly pink, add the tomatoes and reduce the heat
to simmer. Simmer for approximately 5 minutes, or until the turkey is fully
cooked and any liquid is cooked off.

Spread the turkey over the beans and chips. Sprinkle the remaining
ingredients in the order listed.

Bake for approximately 5 minutes, or until the cheese is melted.

PROTEIN POWERED	CARBOHYDRATE CONCENTRATED	FAT FRIENDLY	FREE FOODS
Ground turkey, Mexican cheese	Whole wheat tortillas, pinto beans, crushed tomatoes	Cooking spray	Taco seasoning, jalapeño chile pepper, scallions, cilantro

*Nutrition facts calculated by Menu Magic Personal Chef Software, Version 2.6, 2008,
Kreotek, LLC, Rio Rancho, New Mexico.*

CHRISTINE'S NUTRITION NUGGETS Pinto beans are a good source of iron, with 2 milligrams
per 1/2-cup serving.

Sicilian Chicken Soup

Nutrition facts per serving: 390 calories, 26 grams protein,
51 grams carbohydrates, 7 grams fat SERVES 8

1 pound boneless, skinless chicken breast tenders

Extra virgin olive oil spray

2 cloves garlic, minced

¼ teaspoon ground red pepper

1 teaspoon crushed red-pepper flakes

1 teaspoon garlic salt

1½ cups water

2 boxes (32 ounces each) low-sodium, free range chicken broth

8 ribs celery, diced

½ pound baby carrots, diced

1 white onion, diced

½ cup whole wheat orzo pasta

3 tablespoons commercially prepared pesto

¼ cup fresh lemon juice

½ teaspoon salt

1 teaspoon ground black pepper

½ cup shredded reduced-fat Parmesan cheese

16 slices whole wheat sourdough bread, toasted

Wash and pat dry the chicken, then cut into small cubes. Place in a large bowl and coat with olive oil spray. Add the next 4 ingredients and mix together so that the spices evenly coat the chicken. Set aside.

Bring the water and chicken broth to a boil in a large Dutch oven. Stir in the celery, carrots, and onion and bring to a boil. Cook for 10 minutes. Add the chicken and continue to boil for 5 minutes. Add the orzo and boil for 4 more minutes, or until the chicken is cooked through. Turn off the heat, add the pesto, lemon juice, and salt and pepper, and stir well. Finally add the cheese; stir again.

Serve with 2 slices toast per serving.

PROTEIN POWERED	CARBOHYDRATE CONCENTRATED	FAT FRIENDLY	FREE FOODS
Chicken, Parmesan cheese	Carrots, whole wheat orzo pasta, whole wheat sourdough bread	Extra virgin olive oil, pesto	Herbs, spices, chicken broth, celery, onion, lemon juice

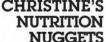
CHRISTINE'S NUTRITION NUGGETS The carrots in this soup provide high amounts of vitamin A (in the form of beta-carotene). Research suggests that vitamin A helps to protect skin and extends its youthful appearance.

Grilled Fat-Free Cheese Sandwich

Nutrition facts per serving: 335 calories, 24 grams protein,
48 grams carbohydrates, 5 grams fat SERVES 1
· ·

1½ slices fat-free Swiss cheese

2 large slices whole wheat bread

1 small tomato, sliced

¼ teaspoon dried oregano

1½ slices fat-free Cheddar cheese

2 teaspoons omega-3 light spread

Place the Swiss on one side of a slice of bread. Then place the tomato slices on top and sprinkle with the oregano.

Follow with the Cheddar and the second piece of bread.

Melt the omega-3 spread in a skillet over medium heat and cook the sandwich for 1 to 2 minutes on each side, or until the cheese is melted and the bread is toasty.

PROTEIN POWERED	CARBOHYDRATE CONCENTRATED	FAT FRIENDLY	FREE FOODS
Fat-free Swiss cheese, fat-free Cheddar cheese	Whole wheat bread	Omega-3 light spread	Tomato, dried oregano

Nutrition facts calculated by Menu Magic Personal Chef Software, Version 2.6, 2008, Kreotek, LLC, Rio Rancho, New Mexico.

CHRISTINE'S NUTRITION NUGGETS Fat-free cheese is a far better option than regular cheese. When shopping for cheese, read the nutrition facts labels, and you will notice that regular cheese has the same amount of fat as it does protein per serving (and sometimes more!). Regular cheese is also high in saturated fats, which are associated with heart disease.

Aioli Chicken Panini

Nutrition facts per serving: 359 calories, 26 grams protein,
43 grams carbohydrates, 9 grams fat SERVES 1
. . . .

1½ tablespoons light mayonnaise

1 teaspoon chopped fresh parsley

1 small tomato, chopped

½ teaspoon minced garlic

1¾ ounces cooked boneless, skinless chicken breast, thinly sliced

2 large slices whole wheat bread

2 tablespoons shredded fat-free mozzarella cheese

Nonstick cooking spray

In a small bowl, mix together the mayonnaise, parsley, tomato, and garlic.

Stir in the chicken and coat well.

Sprinkle one side of one slice of bread with half of the cheese.

Spread the chicken mixture on top and sprinkle with the remaining cheese.

Coat a nonstick pan with cooking spray. Cook the panini over medium heat
for approximately 1 to 2 minutes on each side, or until golden.

PROTEIN POWERED	CARBOHYDRATE CONCENTRATED	FAT FRIENDLY	FREE FOODS
Chicken, fat-free mozzarella cheese	Whole wheat bread	Light mayo, cooking spray	Parsley, tomato, garlic,

*Nutrition facts calculated by Menu Magic Personal Chef Software, Version 2.6, 2008,
Kreotek, LLC, Rio Rancho, New Mexico.*

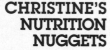 **CHRISTINE'S NUTRITION NUGGETS** Choose whole grain bread instead of multigrain bread. Whole grain is made from 100 percent of the grain kernel, whereas multigrain is made from enriched wheat flour. The key is to look for the word *whole* when shopping for bread.

Bruschetta Chicken Wrap

Nutrition facts per serving: 367 calories, 27 grams protein,
46 grams carbohydrates, 8 grams fat SERVES 1

• •

1 medium tomato, chopped

1 tablespoon chopped fresh basil

1 teaspoon minced garlic

2 tablespoons fat-free balsamic dressing

½ teaspoon extra virgin olive oil

2 ounces cooked boneless, skinless chicken breast, thinly sliced

1 cup fresh spinach

1 large whole wheat tortilla

In a medium bowl, toss the first 7 ingredients together.

Place the mixture in the center of the tortilla. Fold the bottom side in and then fold in the sides.

PROTEIN POWERED	CARBOHYDRATE CONCENTRATED	FAT FRIENDLY	FREE FOODS
Chicken breast	Whole wheat tortilla	Extra virgin olive oil	Tomato, basil, garlic, fat-free dressing, spinach

Nutrition facts calculated by Menu Magic Personal Chef Software, Version 2.6, 2008, Kreotek, LLC, Rio Rancho, New Mexico.

CHRISTINE'S NUTRITION NUGGETS Garlic contains a phytonutrient called allicin, which is known to destroy bad bacteria such as yeast and fungi in the intestines.

No-Fry Chicken Fried Rice

Nutrition facts per serving: 381 calories, 28 grams protein,
45 grams carbohydrates, 10 grams fat SERVES 4

¼ cup low-sodium soy sauce

1 tablespoon oyster sauce

1 tablespoon crushed ginger

1 tablespoon minced garlic

½ cup fat-free, sodium-free
chicken broth

2 teaspoons extra virgin olive oil

1 teaspoon omega-3 light spread

1 cup chopped red cabbage

2 cups broccoli crowns, cut small

1 cup chopped red bell pepper

½ cup chopped scallions

3 cups brown rice, cooked

10 ounces boneless, skinless
chicken breasts, grilled and chopped

2 tablespoons toasted sesame seeds

1 teaspoon crushed red-pepper
flakes

In a small bowl, mix together the soy sauce, oyster sauce, ginger, garlic, and chicken broth and set aside.

In a large wok or skillet, heat the oil and omega-3 spread over medium-high heat. Sauté the vegetables for approximately 2 minutes.

Add the soy mixture, then add the rice and mix well.

When the rice is almost heated, add the chicken and cook until heated through, approximately 3 to 5 minutes.

Transfer to a serving dish and sprinkle with the sesame seeds and pepper flakes.

PROTEIN POWERED	CARBOHYDRATE CONCENTRATED	FAT FRIENDLY	FREE FOODS
Chicken breast	Brown rice	Extra virgin olive oil	Soy sauce, oyster sauce, ginger, chicken broth, red cabbage, broccoli, red bell pepper, scallions, red-pepper flakes

Nutrition facts calculated by Menu Magic Personal Chef Software, Version 2.6, 2008, Kreotek, LLC, Rio Rancho, New Mexico.

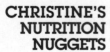

CHRISTINE'S NUTRITION NUGGETS Stir-frying vegetables causes fewer vitamins to be lost than boiling them does. Ginger is an ancient Chinese cure for colds. Fresh ginger might fight viruses by causing the body to sweat out toxins.

Christine's Pasta and Spicy Red Sauce

Nutrition facts per serving: 425 calories, 31 grams protein, 59 grams carbohydrates, 9 grams fat SERVES 4

• •

Nonstick cooking spray

2 teaspoons extra virgin olive oil

2–3 cloves garlic, minced

½ teaspoon crushed red-pepper flakes

½ teaspoon dried Italian seasoning or oregano

½ teaspoon salt

¼ teaspoon ground black pepper

¼ teaspoon ground red pepper

1 medium onion, chopped

1 pound extra-lean ground turkey

1 small green bell pepper, diced

8 ounces sliced mushrooms

1 jar (26 ounces) pasta sauce (I love Classico spicy red pepper)

1 can (16 ounces) diced tomatoes

½ cup reduced-fat Parmesan cheese

1 pound whole wheat spaghetti or your favorite pasta

Note: *Omit the red-pepper flakes if you do not like it spicy.*

Coat a 3-quart rectangular baking dish with cooking spray; set aside. Heat the oil in a large saucepan; sauté the garlic, spices, salt and black pepper, ground red pepper, and onion for 2 minutes. Add the turkey and cook until browned. Next add the bell pepper and mushrooms; sauté for 4 more minutes. Add the pasta sauce and tomatoes and bring to a boil; reduce the heat. Simmer, uncovered, for 15 minutes, stirring occasionally. Stir the cheese into the sauce before serving.

Prepare the pasta according to package directions. For al dente pasta, take 3 minutes off the recommended boiling time.

Serve 1 cup of cooked pasta topped with red sauce per serving.

PROTEIN POWERED	CARBOHYDRATE CONCENTRATED	FAT FRIENDLY	FREE FOODS
Extra-lean ground turkey	Whole wheat pasta	Extra virgin olive oil	Mushrooms, garlic, spices, onion, bell pepper, tomatoes

Creamy Lemon Basil Chicken Linguine

Nutrition facts per serving: 386 calories, 31 grams protein,
54 grams carbohydrates, 5 grams fat SERVES 4

½ cup low-fat sour cream

½ cup whole milk

½ cup fat-free, sodium-free
chicken broth

2 tablespoons lemon juice

1½ teaspoons minced garlic

1 cup fresh basil

1 medium lemon, peeled and sliced
(grate the peel)

¼ teaspoon crushed red-pepper
flakes

8 ounces whole wheat linguine

12 ounces boneless, skinless
chicken breasts, cut into ½" strips

Salt

Ground black pepper

Nonstick cooking spray

Basil sprigs, for garnish

In a medium bowl, combine the sour cream, milk, chicken broth, lemon juice, and garlic.

Chop the basil in a food processor.

Turn on the processor and slowly add the liquid mixture. Turn off the processor as soon as the bowl is empty.

Transfer to a saucepan. Stir in the lemon peel and pepper flakes, then set aside.

Cook the linguine according to package directions.

Season the chicken with salt and black pepper. Spray a skillet with cooking spray, and heat on medium high. Brown the chicken on each side for 3 to 4 minutes, or until cooked through.

When the chicken and linguine are cooked, heat the sauce for 3 to 5 minutes over medium-low heat. Do not bring to a boil.

Toss together the sauce, linguine, and chicken. Garnish with the lemon slices and basil sprigs.

PROTEIN POWERED	CARBOHYDRATE CONCENTRATED	FAT FRIENDLY	FREE FOODS
Chicken breasts, milk	Whole wheat linguine	Cooking spray	Chicken broth, lemon juice, herbs, spices

Nutrition facts calculated by Menu Magic Personal Chef Software, Version 2.6, 2008, Kreotek, LLC, Rio Rancho, New Mexico.

Mediterranean Shrimp Pasta

Nutrition facts per serving: 399 calories, 30 grams protein,
48 grams carbohydrates, 10 grams fat SERVES 4

8 ounces brown rice fusilli or spiral pasta

4 medium tomatoes, seeded and chopped

4 cups raw spinach

2 tablespoons extra virgin olive oil

¼ teaspoon salt

¼ teaspoon ground black pepper

1 tablespoon minced garlic

1 pound raw shrimp, peeled and deveined

1 tablespoon lemon juice

¼ cup chopped fresh basil

Peel of 1 lemon, grated

Cook the pasta according to package directions.

In a large skillet over medium-high heat, sauté the tomatoes and spinach in the olive oil with the salt, pepper, and garlic.

When the spinach has started to wilt, add the shrimp, lemon juice, and basil, and cook until the shrimp are pink.

Toss with the pasta and sprinkle with the lemon peel.

PROTEIN POWERED	CARBOHYDRATE CONCENTRATED	FAT FRIENDLY	FREE FOODS
Shrimp	Brown rice pasta	Extra virgin olive oil	Tomatoes, spinach, garlic, lemon, basil

Nutrition facts calculated by Menu Magic Personal Chef Software, Version 2.6, 2008, Kreotek, LLC, Rio Rancho, New Mexico.

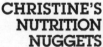

CHRISTINE'S NUTRITION NUGGETS Shrimp are a fantastic source of lean protein; however, if you have high cholesterol, you should avoid shrimp and use clams or chicken breast. Shrimp are a little high in cholesterol and only need to be avoided by people who have high cholesterol.

Christine's Born-Again Lasagna

Nutrition facts per serving: 467 calories, 34 grams protein,
61 grams carbohydrates, 8 grams fat SERVES 12

• •

Nonstick cooking spray

2 teaspoons extra virgin olive oil

2–3 cloves garlic, minced

$\frac{1}{2}$ teaspoon crushed red-pepper flakes

$\frac{1}{2}$ teaspoon dried Italian seasoning or oregano

$\frac{1}{4}$ teaspoon ground black pepper

$\frac{1}{4}$ teaspoon ground red pepper

$\frac{1}{2}$ teaspoon salt

1 medium onion, chopped

1 pound extra-lean ground turkey

1 small green bell pepper, diced

8 ounces sliced mushrooms

1 jar (26 ounces) pasta sauce (I love Classico spicy red pepper)

1 can (16 ounces) diced tomatoes

15 ounces fat-free ricotta cheese (available at Whole Foods Market)

2 tablespoons chopped fresh parsley + extra for garnish

2 egg whites, lightly beaten

9 no-boil whole wheat lasagna noodles

1 cup shredded fat-free mozzarella

1 cup part-skim mozzarella

$\frac{1}{2}$ cup reduced-fat Parmesan cheese

12 slices sourdough bread

Coat a 3-quart rectangular baking dish with cooking spray; set aside. Heat the oil in a large saucepan; sauté the garlic, spices, salt, and onion for 2 minutes. Add the turkey and cook until browned. Next add the bell pepper and mushrooms; sauté for 4 more minutes. Add the pasta sauce and tomatoes and bring to a boil; reduce the heat. Simmer, uncovered, for 15 minutes, stirring occasionally.

Preheat the oven to 375°F. In a medium bowl, combine the ricotta, parsley, and egg until smooth, set aside. Cover the bottom of the prepared baking dish with half of the lasagna noodles; then spread half of the ricotta mixture on top, followed by half of the meat sauce and a light layer of mozzarella cheese. Repeat the layering process.

Cover and bake for 40 minutes. Uncover. Sprinkle with the Parmesan and bake for 10 minutes. Let stand for 10 minutes before serving. Garnish with parsley.

PROTEIN POWERED	CARBOHYDRATE CONCENTRATED	FAT FRIENDLY	FREE FOODS
Extra-lean ground turkey, fat-free ricotta, fat-free mozzarella	Whole wheat lasagna noodles, pasta sauce, tomatoes	Extra virgin olive oil, part-skim mozzarella	Herbs, spices, onion, mushrooms, bell pepper

Wasabi Sesame Salmon with Brown Rice Noodles

Nutrition facts per serving: 400 calories, 25 grams protein,
48 grams carbohydrates, 12 grams fat SERVES 4

. . . .

SALMON

Nonstick cooking spray

15 ounces wild salmon,
cut into 4 pieces

Pinch of salt

Pinch of ground black pepper

¼ cup light mayonnaise

1 tablespoon wasabi

1 tablespoon black sesame seeds

NOODLES

8 ounces brown rice spaghetti

1 cup shredded carrots

¼ cup low-sodium soy sauce

¼ cup fat-free, sodium-free
chicken broth

½ teaspoon Sriracha chili sauce

¼ cup chopped scallions

TO MAKE THE SALMON:

Preheat the oven to 375°F. Spray a baking pan with cooking spray. Place the salmon on the pan and season with the salt and pepper.

Mix the mayonnaise and wasabi together and brush evenly on the salmon. Sprinkle with the sesame seeds. Bake for 7 to 10 minutes, or until the salmon is opaque.

TO MAKE THE NOODLES:

Cook the spaghetti according to package directions. One minute before draining, add the carrots.

Mix the soy sauce, broth, and chili sauce together. Stir the sauce into the drained noodles. Top with the scallions.

PROTEIN POWERED	CARBOHYDRATE CONCENTRATED	FAT FRIENDLY	FREE FOODS
Salmon	Brown rice spaghetti, carrots	Light mayonnaise, sesame seeds	Wasabi, soy sauce, chicken broth, chili sauce, scallions

Nutrition facts calculated by Menu Magic Personal Chef Software, Version 2.6, 2008, Kreotek, LLC, Rio Rancho, New Mexico.

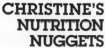 **CHRISTINE'S NUTRITION NUGGETS** Brown rice noodles offer an excellent alternative for people who suffer from celiac disease, a wheat gluten allergy. They also pack in fiber, which is known to help stabilize blood sugar levels.

Sugar and Spice Salmon with Barbecue Sweet Potatoes

Nutrition facts per serving: 367 calories, 24 grams protein, 51 grams carbohydrates, 7 grams fat SERVES 4

SALMON

Nonstick cooking spray

2 tablespoons brown sugar

2 teaspoons chili powder

1 teaspoon cumin

1 teaspoon paprika

$\frac{1}{2}$ teaspoon salt

$\frac{1}{2}$ teaspoon ground black pepper

$\frac{1}{4}$ teaspoon ground red pepper

1 pound wild salmon, cut in 4 pieces

SWEET POTATOES

$\frac{1}{4}$ cup barbecue sauce

$\frac{1}{4}$ cup fat-free, sodium-free chicken broth

4 medium sweet potatoes, cut into $\frac{1}{4}$" rounds

Nonstick cooking spray

TO MAKE THE SALMON:

Preheat the oven to 375ºF. Spray a baking pan with cooking spray.

In a small bowl, mix all the dry ingredients together. Dust the top of each piece of salmon with the spice mix, then place in the prepared baking pan. Bake for 7 to 10 minutes, or until the salmon is opaque.

TO MAKE THE SWEET POTATOES:

Mix the barbecue sauce and broth together well. Gently stir the sweet potatoes in the sauce to coat well. Remove the sweet potato slices and place on a baking sheet coated with cooking spray. Keep the potatoes in a single layer and use a second baking sheet if needed. Bake for 15 minutes at 375ºF.

PROTEIN POWERED	CARBOHYDRATE CONCENTRATED	FAT FRIENDLY	FREE FOODS
Salmon	Barbecue sauce, sweet potatoes	Heart-healthy fat in the salmon; cooking spray	Spices, chicken broth

Nutrition facts calculated by Menu Magic Personal Chef Software, Version 2.6, 2008, Kreotek, LLC, Rio Rancho, New Mexico.

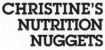

CHRISTINE'S NUTRITION NUGGETS Adding hot spices to your meals can help curb hunger, according to a study in the *British Journal of Nutrition*. Additionally, scientists at the State University of New York at Buffalo found that capsaicin (a compound found in chile peppers) triggers your brain to release feel-good endorphins.

Citrus Tilapia

Nutrition facts per serving: 385 calories, 27 grams protein, 47 grams carbohydrates, 10 grams fat SERVES 4

. . . .

1 pound Roma tomatoes, diced

Juice and grated peel of 1 orange

¼ cup minced green olives

2 cups water

Salt

1½ cups quinoa, uncooked

2 tablespoons extra virgin olive oil, divided

Nonstick cooking spray

1 pound tilapia

Ground black pepper to taste

Preheat the oven to 375ºF.

In a medium sauté pan, combine the tomatoes, orange juice, orange peel, olives, and 1 tablespoon of the oil. Cook for 4 minutes, then set aside.

In a medium saucepan, bring the water to a boil with a pinch of salt. Add the quinoa and 1 tablespoon of the oil; cover and cook for 2 minutes. Turn off the heat; let stand until the quinoa absorbs all of the liquid (about 5 minutes).

Spray a roasting pan with cooking spray, season the tilapia with salt and pepper, and bake for 10 minutes.

Layer each plate with quinoa, then top with tilapia and finally with tomato mixture.

PROTEIN POWERED	CARBOHYDRATE CONCENTRATED	FAT FRIENDLY	FREE FOODS
Tilapia	Orange juice, quinoa	Green olives, extra virgin olive oil	Roma tomatoes, orange peel

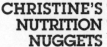 **CHRISTINE'S NUTRITION NUGGETS** Green olives and olive oil contain high amounts of compounds deemed to be anticancer agents, according to the *European Journal of Cancer Prevention*.

Coconut Curry Sea Bass over Red Lentils

Nutrition facts per serving: 344 calories, 25 grams protein,
42 grams carbohydrates, 9 grams fat SERVES 4

Nonstick cooking spray

4 banana leaves or string
for tying up sea bass

1 leek

1 small red bell pepper

1 small yellow bell pepper

1 small orange bell pepper

¼ teaspoon yellow curry powder

¼ cup coconut flakes

12 ounces sea bass,
cut into 4 fillets

¾ cup light coconut milk

1 tablespoon agave nectar

1 pound dried red lentils

Preheat the oven to 400°F. Cover a medium-size baking sheet with foil and spray with cooking spray.

Cut off the edges of the banana leaves, if using, so that you have long strips of banana leaf to use as ties. If you do not have banana leaves, use string.

Slice the leek and peppers. In a shallow bowl, combine the curry and coconut. Roll all sides of the fish in the coconut mixture to lightly coat.

Place one piece of fish, some of the leek slices, and some pepper slices in a banana leaf. Put 1 tablespoon of coconut milk and a drop of agave nectar on each piece of fish and roll up each fish fillet.

Tie two banana leaf strips or string around each fish fillet, place onto the prepared baking sheet, and bake for 20 minutes.

While the fish is baking, prepare the lentils according to the package directions. While the lentils are cooking, place any extra vegetables, coconut milk, and 1 teaspoon of agave nectar in a medium saucepan, and cook over medium heat for 5 minutes, stirring occasionally.

When the fish flakes easily, place each fillet on top of 1 cup of cooked lentils and top with the coconut curry veggie sauce.

PROTEIN POWERED	CARBOHYDRATE CONCENTRATED	FAT FRIENDLY	FREE FOODS
Sea bass	Red lentils	Light coconut milk, coconut flakes	Banana leaves, curry, peppers

Cilantro Lime Sea Bass

Nutrition facts per serving: 338 calories, 25 grams protein,
47 grams carbohydrates, 5 grams fat SERVES 4

· ·

4 fillets fresh sea bass (3 ounces each)

Juice of 2 limes

½ bunch fresh cilantro, chopped

Salt and ground black pepper to taste

2 tablespoons extra virgin olive oil

2 cups water

¼ teaspoon turmeric

½ cup raisins

1 tablespoon chopped fresh ginger

1 cup dry (uncooked) couscous

Note: *For a kick-start meal, swap the raisin couscous for brown rice.*

Place the sea bass in a roasting pan and add the lime juice, cilantro, salt, and
pepper. Cover with plastic wrap and marinate for 1 hour in the refrigerator.

Preheat the oven to 350°F. While the fish is marinating, prepare the
couscous. Bring the oil, water, a pinch of salt, the turmeric, raisins, and ginger
to a boil; add the couscous. Cover and simmer for approximately 5 minutes or
until the water is absorbed.

Uncover the sea bass and cook for 15 minutes or until the fish flakes easily.

Serve the sea bass over the couscous.

PROTEIN POWERED	CARBOHYDRATE CONCENTRATED	FAT FRIENDLY	FREE FOODS
Sea bass	Couscous, raisins	Extra virgin olive oil	Limes, cilantro, turmeric, ginger

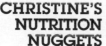 **CHRISTINE'S NUTRITION NUGGETS** Turmeric is a potent antioxidant with anti-inflammatory properties. Some evidence suggests that turmeric has the potential to act as an anticancer agent.

Cajun-Style Grilled Shrimp

Nutrition facts per serving: 410 calories, 28 grams protein,
50 grams carbohydrates, 11 grams fat SERVES 4

1 pound peeled and deveined medium shrimp

2 tablespoons extra virgin olive oil

Juice of 2 lemons

4 tablespoons Cajun spice, such as Emeril's

Salt and ground black pepper to taste

2 cups water

1¼ cups uncooked brown rice

Nonstick cooking spray

1 lemon, cut into 4 pieces

In a shallow dish, marinate the shrimp with the olive oil, lemon juice, Cajun spice, and salt and pepper for 20 minutes at room temperature.

While the shrimp is marinating, prepare the rice. Bring the water to a boil; add the rice, cover, and simmer for approximately 17 to 20 minutes or until the water is absorbed.

Warm a sauté pan over medium heat. Remove from the heat, spray with cooking spray, and return to the heat. Add the shrimp and cook for 2 minutes on each side, or until the shrimp are pink.

Serve with the rice and garnish with the lemon.

PROTEIN POWERED	CARBOHYDRATE CONCENTRATED	FAT FRIENDLY	FREE FOODS
Shrimp	Brown rice	Extra virgin olive oil	Lemon, Cajun spice, salt, pepper

CHRISTINE'S NUTRITION NUGGETS Shrimp are high in vitamin D, which is important for increasing calcium absorption and thus increasing bone growth. Vitamin D has been shown to help prevent certain cancers, heart disease, diabetes, and osteoarthritis. The recommended daily adequate intake for adults is 200 International Units (IU). This meal provides 172 IU of vitamin D.

Apricot Glazed Chicken with Spicy Quinoa

Nutrition facts per serving: 386 calories, 28 grams protein, 47 grams carbohydrates, 9 grams fat SERVES 4

CHICKEN

Nonstick cooking spray

12 ounces boneless, skinless chicken breasts

1/3 cup fat-free, sodium-free chicken broth

1/3 cup sugar-free apricot preserves

1 1/2 teaspoons Dijon mustard

3/4 teaspoon Worcestershire sauce

1 1/2 tablespoons low-cal French dressing

1/2 teaspoon garlic powder

QUINOA

1 1/2 cups quinoa

1 tablespoon extra virgin olive oil

1/3 cup chopped celery

1/3 cup chopped red bell pepper

1/4 cup chopped onion

1 teaspoon paprika

1/4 teaspoon ground red pepper

1/2 teaspoon salt

1/4 teaspoon ground black pepper

TO MAKE THE CHICKEN:

Coat a skillet with cooking spray and place over medium-high heat. Add the chicken and cook until browned. Transfer to a sheet pan and set aside.

Combine the next 6 ingredients in a medium saucepan over medium heat. When the ingredients are mixed well, lower the heat and simmer for approximately 5 minutes, or until the sauce is slightly thickened.

Spoon the sauce over the chicken and bake at 350ºF for approximately 8 to 12 minutes, or until the chicken is cooked through.

TO MAKE THE QUINOA:

Cook the quinoa according to the package directions, adding the oil, celery, bell pepper, and onion to the quinoa before cooking.

When the quinoa is cooked, stir in the paprika, ground red pepper, salt, and black pepper.

PROTEIN POWERED	CARBOHYDRATE CONCENTRATED	FAT FRIENDLY	FREE FOODS
Chicken	Quinoa, apricot preserves	Extra virgin olive oil, cooking spray, French dressing	Chicken broth, Dijon mustard, Worcestershire sauce, spices, celery, red bell pepper, onion

Sicilian-Style Chicken and Rice

Nutrition facts per serving: 414 calories, 33 grams protein, 56 grams carbohydrates, 6 grams fat SERVES 12

Nonstick cooking spray

2 tablespoons extra virgin olive oil

2 cloves garlic, minced

1/2 teaspoon oregano

1/4 teaspoon ground red pepper

1/4 teaspoon salt

1/4 teaspoon ground black pepper

3 pounds boneless, skinless chicken breast tenders

1 cup whole wheat flour

1 large white onion, chopped

1 pound large white mushrooms, sliced

3 medium green bell peppers, thinly sliced

3 cups water

1 can (15 ounces) tomato sauce

4 cups brown rice, cooked

Coat the bottom of a 6-quart Dutch oven with cooking spray. Place the olive oil on the bottom of the pot and add the garlic, oregano, red pepper, salt, and black pepper. Sauté for 1 to 2 minutes.

Wash and pat dry the chicken, then coat with the flour. Add one-quarter of the onion and the floured chicken to the Dutch oven and cook until the meat is no longer pink. Add the mushrooms and bell peppers and the remaining onion and sauté another 5 minutes.

Add the water and tomato sauce. Stir several times to keep the ingredients from sticking to the bottom of the pot. Cook on medium low for 1 hour and 15 minutes.

PROTEIN POWERED	CARBOHYDRATE CONCENTRATED	FAT FRIENDLY	FREE FOODS
Chicken breast	Brown rice, whole wheat flour, tomato sauce	Extra virgin olive oil	Mushrooms, bell peppers, onion, garlic, ground red pepper

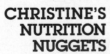

CHRISTINE'S NUTRITION NUGGETS Mushrooms are loaded with biotin, and this meal provides 6 micrograms of biotin per serving. Biotin in its physiologically active form attaches to enzymes that are required for the synthesis of fatty acids.

Balsamic Herb Chicken with French Lentils

Nutrition facts per serving: 386 calories, 32 grams protein, 46 grams carbohydrates, 8 grams fat SERVES 4

CHICKEN

$\frac{1}{2}$ cup balsamic vinegar

11 ounces boneless, skinless chicken breast tenders

$\frac{1}{2}$ teaspoon salt

$\frac{1}{2}$ teaspoon ground black pepper

1 tablespoon Herbes de Provence

Nonstick cooking spray

4 fresh rosemary sprigs

4 fresh lavender sprigs (optional)

LENTILS

1 tablespoon extra virgin olive oil

$\frac{1}{2}$ cup chopped onion

1 cup sliced mushrooms

$\frac{1}{4}$ cup vegetable broth

2 tablespoons Dijon mustard

1 tablespoon minced garlic

1 teaspoon thyme

2 cups chopped savoy cabbage

2 cups canned lentils, rinsed and drained

$1\frac{1}{2}$ cups pearl barley, cooked

Salt and ground black pepper

1 tablespoon sliced almonds, toasted

TO MAKE THE CHICKEN:

In a small saucepan over low heat, simmer the vinegar until thick and syrupy.

Season the chicken with the salt and pepper, and coat it with the herbs. Spray a large skillet with cooking spray. Over medium-high heat, cook the chicken about 3 to 4 minutes on each side, or until cooked through. Transfer to a serving dish and drizzle with the balsamic reduction. Garnish with the rosemary and lavender (if desired).

TO MAKE THE LENTILS:

Warm the oil over medium heat in a large skillet. Add the onion and cook until slightly soft, then stir in the mushrooms. When the mushrooms are slightly soft, stir in the broth, mustard, garlic, and thyme. Let simmer until the mushrooms are just cooked through.

Add the cabbage, lentils, and barley, and cook until heated throughout. Season with salt and pepper to taste. Sprinkle with the almonds.

PROTEIN POWERED	CARBOHYDRATE CONCENTRATED	FAT FRIENDLY	FREE FOODS
Chicken	Lentils (have both protein and carbs), pearl barley	Cooking spray, extra virgin olive oil, almonds	Herbs, spices, balsamic vinegar, onion, mushrooms, Dijon mustard, cabbage

Nutrition facts calculated by Menu Magic Personal Chef Software, Version 2.6, 2008, Kreotek, LLC, Rio Rancho, New Mexico.

Mushroom and Artichoke Chicken Scaloppine

Nutrition facts per serving: 393 calories, 29 grams protein, 48 grams carbohydrates, 9 grams fat SERVES 4

. . . .

CHICKEN SCALOPPINE

12 ounces boneless, skinless chicken cutlets

1/2 teaspoon salt, divided

1/2 teaspoon ground black pepper, divided

2 tablespoons extra virgin olive oil

1/2 cup dry white wine

1 1/2 cups sliced mushrooms

1/2 cup chopped shallots

1 tablespoon omega-3 light spread

1 teaspoon thyme

1/2 cup fat-free, sodium-free chicken broth

1 tablespoon minced garlic

1 1/2 cups canned artichoke hearts in water, quartered

2 tablespoons cornstarch

2 tablespoons water

1 tablespoon chopped fresh parsley

WILD RICE

3 cups cooked wild rice

Juice and grated peel of 1 medium lemon

TO MAKE THE CHICKEN:

Season the chicken with half of the salt and half of the pepper. Using the oil as needed, brown each side of the chicken in a large skillet until cooked through. Remove the chicken and keep warm. Deglaze the pan with the wine, scraping the bottom until clean. Strain and set the liquid aside.

Meanwhile, in a skillet, sauté the mushrooms and shallots in the omega-3 spread with the remaining salt and pepper, and the thyme. After 3 minutes, add the broth and garlic. Simmer for another 5 minutes, or until the mushrooms are soft. Add the artichokes and cook for 1 minute more. Stir in the liquid from the deglazed pan.

In a small bowl, mix the cornstarch and water. Slowly add to the mushrooms while stirring. Cook until slightly thickened.

Stir the lemon juice and peel into the wild rice and serve with the chicken. Pour the sauce over the chicken and sprinkle with parsley.

PROTEIN POWERED	CARBOHYDRATE CONCENTRATED	FAT FRIENDLY	FREE FOODS
Chicken breast	Wild rice, artichoke hearts	Extra virgin olive oil, omega-3 light spread	Herbs, mushrooms, shallots, chicken broth, cornstarch, lemon

Nutrition facts calculated by Menu Magic Personal Chef Software, Version 2.6, 2008, Kreotek, LLC, Rio Rancho, New Mexico.

Chicken Kebabs
on Lemon Grass Skewers

Nutrition facts per serving: 338 calories, 25 grams protein,
47 grams carbohydrates, 5 grams fat SERVES 4
. . . .

1 pound chicken breasts, cut into
8 pieces (use 2 pieces per kebab)

1 onion, cut into cubes

1 red bell pepper, cut into squares

¼ cup teriyaki sauce

1 tablespoon sesame oil

4 cups water

2 cups jasmine rice

4 lemon grass sticks
(for use as skewers)

Olive oil cooking spray

2 lemons

In a large plastic bag, marinate the chicken, onion, and pepper in the teriyaki
sauce and sesame oil for 20 minutes at room temperature.

While the chicken marinates, prepare the rice. Bring the water to a boil; add
the rice, cover, and simmer for 20 minutes or until the water is absorbed.

Build your kebabs by alternating the chicken, onion, and pepper on each
lemon grass skewer. Spray the kebabs with olive oil cooking spray.

Grill until the chicken is cooked through, about 5 minutes on each side.

Garnish with half of a lemon on each plate.

PROTEIN POWERED	CARBOHYDRATE CONCENTRATED	FAT FRIENDLY	FREE FOODS
Chicken breast	Jasmine rice	Sesame oil, cooking spray	Lemon grass sticks, onion, red bell pepper, lemons

CHRISTINE'S NUTRITION NUGGETS Lemon grass has been shown to reduce oxidative stress caused by free radical damage. Additionally, the aroma of lemon grass is known to have a calming effect on the central nervous system.

Grilled Chicken Fajitas with Mango Salsa

Nutrition facts per serving: 417 calories, 30 grams protein, 56 grams carbohydrates, 8 grams fat SERVES 4

. . . .

¼ cup lime juice

1 teaspoon chili powder

1 teaspoon cumin

1 teaspoon minced garlic

1 teaspoon oregano

¼ teaspoon crushed red-pepper flakes

14 ounces boneless, skinless chicken breasts, cut into ¾"-wide strips

2 cups sliced red bell peppers (cut into ½" strips)

2 cups sliced onions (cut into ½" strips)

1 cup fresh salsa

½ medium mango, chopped

½ medium avocado, chopped

½ teaspoon salt

½ teaspoon ground black pepper

High-heat nonstick cooking spray

8 corn tortillas

2 limes, sliced

¼ cup fat-free sour cream

Preheat a grill pan or outdoor grill. Whisk the first 6 ingredients together in a small bowl. Divide into 2 large plastic bags. Add the chicken to one bag and the peppers and onions to the other. Shake the bags to coat thoroughly. Let marinate for at least ½ hour.

In a medium bowl, combine the salsa, mango, and avocado and set aside.

Season the chicken and vegetables with the salt and black pepper. Spray the grill with the cooking spray.

Grill the chicken until cooked through, approximately 4 minutes on each side. Grill the vegetables until brown, 10 to 15 minutes, turning frequently.

Wrap the tortillas in foil and place on the grill until warmed, 3 to 5 minutes.

Stuff the tortillas with the chicken, peppers, and onion, and top with the mango salsa. Garnish with the lime slices and serve with the sour cream.

PROTEIN POWERED	CARBOHYDRATE CONCENTRATED	FAT FRIENDLY	FREE FOODS
Chicken breast	Corn tortillas, mango	Cooking spray, avocado	Lime juice, herbs, spices, bell peppers, onions, salsa, fat-free sour cream

Nutrition facts calculated by Menu Magic Personal Chef Software, Version 2.6, 2008, Kreotek, LLC, Rio Rancho, New Mexico.

Tex-Mex Chicken with Chipotle Sauce

Nutrition facts per serving: 345 calories, 23 grams protein,
53 grams carbohydrates, 9 grams fat SERVES 6

. . . .

TEX-MEX CHICKEN

1 pound skinless, boneless chicken breasts

Juice of 2 limes

2 tablespoons extra virgin olive oil

1 teaspoon chipotle adobo sauce (from can)

Nonstick cooking spray

1 yellow onion, thinly julienned

1 yellow bell pepper, thinly julienned

1 red bell pepper, thinly julienned

PICO DE GALLO

½ pound Roma tomatoes, chopped

½ bunch fresh cilantro, chopped

Salt and ground black pepper to taste

1 jalapeño chile pepper, chopped, seeds removed

2 medium avocados

BLACK BEAN SUCCOTASH

24 ounces frozen corn, prepared according to package directions

3 cups canned, low-sodium organic black beans

TO MAKE THE TEX-MEX CHICKEN:

Marinate the chicken breasts with the lime juice, oil, and adobo sauce for a minimum of 1 hour in the refrigerator, covered with plastic wrap.

Grill the chicken over medium heat until cooked through, about 6 minutes on each side.

Coat a medium sauté pan with cooking spray and sauté the onion and peppers for 5 minutes. Add the cooked chicken and set aside.

TO MAKE THE PICO DE GALLO:

In a bowl, combine the tomatoes, cilantro, salt, black pepper, and jalapeño.

Peel the avocados and cut each into thin slices.

Arrange the chicken on four plates, cover with the pico de gallo and one-third of an avocado, and serve with ½ cup corn and ½ cup black beans. If you are not on the kick-start program, you may also serve with 3 small corn tortillas per person.

PROTEIN POWERED	CARBOHYDRATE CONCENTRATED	FAT FRIENDLY	FREE FOODS
Chicken breast	Black beans, corn	Olive oil, avocado	Limes, chipotle adobo sauce, bell pepper, onion, Roma tomatoes, cilantro, jalapeño chile pepper

Baked Turkey Chimichanga

Nutrition facts per serving: 392 calories, 27 grams protein,
50 grams carbohydrates, 9 grams fat SERVES 2

5 ounces extra-lean ground turkey

1 pinch each of salt and ground black pepper

$\frac{1}{2}$ cup fresh salsa

$\frac{2}{3}$ cup fat-free refried black beans with jalapeño chile peppers

2 tablespoons canned diced green chile peppers

Nonstick cooking spray

2 large whole wheat tortillas

$\frac{1}{4}$ cup fat-free sour cream

Preheat the oven to 375ºF.

Cook the turkey with the salt and pepper in a nonstick pan until almost done.

Add the salsa, beans, and chile peppers and cook off any liquid from the salsa.

Spray a baking sheet with cooking spray and lay the tortillas out flat.

Pour half of the turkey mixture into the center of each tortilla, and roll up like a burrito.

Bake for approximately 10 minutes or until slightly crispy.

Serve with the sour cream.

PROTEIN POWERED	CARBOHYDRATE CONCENTRATED	FAT FRIENDLY	FREE FOODS
Ground turkey	Refried black beans, whole wheat tortillas	Cooking spray	Salsa, green chile peppers, fat-free sour cream

Nutrition facts calculated by Menu Magic Personal Chef Software, Version 2.6, 2008, Kreotek, LLC, Rio Rancho, New Mexico.

CHRISTINE'S NUTRITION NUGGETS Black beans are an excellent natural PC Combo food. Half a cup of refried black beans contains 6 grams of protein, 18 grams of carbohydrates, 7 grams of fiber, and 1.5 grams of fat. They are a fantastic food when it comes to keeping blood sugar levels stable.

Christine's Enchiladas

Nutrition facts per serving: 372 calories, 28 grams protein, 54 grams carbohydrates, 7 grams fat SERVES 8

. . . .

1 tablespoon extra virgin olive oil

2 cloves garlic, minced

1 teaspoon crushed red-pepper flakes

½ teaspoon ground red pepper

1 teaspoon garlic salt

1 medium white onion, diced

1 pound extra-lean ground turkey

1 can (19 ounces) enchilada sauce

1 can (3.8 ounces) sliced black olives

¼ cup chopped fresh cilantro + additional for garnish

1 can (4 ounces) diced green chile peppers

2 cups shredded fat-free Cheddar cheese

16 white corn tortillas (6" diameter)

4 cups cooked brown rice

Salsa

Fat-free sour cream (optional)

Preheat the oven to 350°F. Place the first 5 ingredients in an extra-large, deep skillet and sauté for 1 to 2 minutes. Add one-quarter of the onion and all of the turkey. Cook until the turkey is completely browned.

Warm the enchilada sauce in a medium saucepan on low for 3 to 5 minutes. While the sauce is warming, in a large mixing bowl, combine the turkey mixture, the remaining onion, and the olives, cilantro, chile peppers, and Cheddar. Set aside.

Coat a 13" × 9" glass baking dish with cooking spray. Spread ¾ cup of the enchilada sauce over the bottom of the baking dish. Then, using a set of tongs, take one tortilla at a time and carefully cover both sides with the sauce. Place ⅓ cup of enchilada mixture into each wet tortilla and roll up. Place each enchilada seam side down into the baking dish.

Once all 16 enchiladas are firmly placed into the baking dish, pour the remaining enchilada sauce over the entire dish of uncooked enchiladas. Cover with foil and bake for 20 minutes. Serve with ½ cup steamed rice, salsa, and fat-free sour cream (if desired), and garnish with extra cilantro.

PROTEIN POWERED	CARBOHYDRATE CONCENTRATED	FAT FRIENDLY	FREE FOODS
Extra-lean ground turkey, fat-free cheese	Rice, enchilada sauce, white corn tortillas	Extra virgin olive oil, black olives	Cilantro, onion, green chile peppers, garlic, red-pepper flakes, spices, salsa, fat-free sour cream

Christine's Favorite Steak with Mushroom Sauce

Nutrition facts per serving: 360 calories, 27 grams protein, 47 grams carbohydrates, 5 grams fat SERVES 4

. . . .

BEEF

½ teaspoon each salt and ground black pepper

1 teaspoon chopped fresh thyme

½ teaspoon chopped fresh rosemary

4 cloves garlic, minced

4 organic top sirloin steaks (3 ounces each)

Cooking spray

SAUCE

1 teaspoon extra virgin olive oil

½ teaspoon fresh thyme

1 package (8 ounces) presliced mushrooms (baby bellas or shiitake)

4 cloves garlic, minced

½ cup organic chicken broth

½ cup Chardonnay

1 tablespoon water

1 teaspoon cornstarch

HERBED MASHED POTATOES

2½ large potatoes

⅔ cup organic chicken broth

1 teaspoon each freshly chopped thyme, chives, and parsley

2 cloves garlic, minced

2 tablespoons low-fat sour cream

Salt and ground black pepper

Note: *If you don't have time to make mashed potatoes, you can substitute with ¾ cup cooked brown rice per serving.*

TO MAKE THE BEEF:

Preheat the oven to 450°F.

Combine the first 5 ingredients. Coat both sides of the steaks with cooking spray; rub steaks evenly with the thyme mixture. Place steaks on the rack of a broiler or roasting pan coated with cooking spray; bake for 8 minutes on each side, or until a thermometer inserted in the center registers 145°F for medium-rare, 160°F for medium, or 165°F for well-done. Remove from the oven; keep warm.

TO MAKE THE SAUCE:

While the steaks are cooking, heat the oil in a large nonstick sauté pan over medium heat. Add the thyme, mushrooms, and garlic; cook 5 minutes or until the mushrooms are tender. Add the broth and wine; bring to a boil. Cook until reduced by half (about 10 minutes).

Combine the water and cornstarch in a small bowl, stirring with a whisk. Add the cornstarch mixture to the pan; bring to a boil. Cook 1 minute or until slightly thickened, stirring constantly. Serve ¼ cup of the sauce with each steak.

TO MAKE THE POTATOES:

Peel the potatoes and cut them in half. Place them in a pot of cold water and cover. Bring to a boil over high heat and simmer until the potatoes are tender when pricked with a fork, about 30 minutes. Drain.

Bring the chicken broth to a boil, then turn down to simmer. Mash the potatoes and combine with the broth, herbs, garlic, and sour cream. Add salt and pepper to taste.

PROTEIN POWERED	CARBOHYDRATE CONCENTRATED	FAT FRIENDLY	FREE FOODS
Sirloin steak	Potatoes or brown rice	Extra virgin olive oil	Mushrooms, garlic, rosemary, thyme, cornstarch, broth

California Fruit Kebabs

Nutrition facts per serving: 313 calories, 27 grams protein, 46 grams carbohydrates, 4 grams fat SERVES 4

8 cubes (1" each) watermelon

8 cubes (1" each) honeydew melon

8 cubes (1" each) cantaloupe

8 large strawberries, stemmed

4 tablespoons orange blossom honey

3 tablespoons chopped fresh mint

4 lemon grass sticks to use as skewers

32 ounces (4 containers) 0% plain Greek yogurt

4 tablespoons slivered almonds

4 whole mint leaves

In a large bowl, mix the fruit together and cover with the honey and chopped mint. Marinate for 20 minutes in the refrigerator.

Assemble the kebabs by alternating the fruit on the lemon grass sticks.

Grill over medium heat for 2 minutes on each side.

Serve with the yogurt in individual bowls for dipping. Garnish the yogurt with the almonds and mint leaves.

PROTEIN POWERED	CARBOHYDRATE CONCENTRATED	FAT FRIENDLY	FREE FOODS
Greek yogurt	Watermelon, honeydew, cantaloupe, strawberries, honey	Slivered almonds	Mint

CHRISTINE'S NUTRITION NUGGETS One serving of these delicious fruit kebabs offers 48 percent of the recommended daily intake (RDI) of vitamin A, which is important for excellent vision and skin. You will also get 92 percent RDI of vitamin C, which enhances collagen production and protects against free radical damage.

Low-Fat, Low-Sugar Pumpkin Bread

Nutrition facts per serving: 196 calories, 5 grams protein,
44 grams carbohydrates, 1 gram fat SERVES 8

Nonstick cooking spray

1 cup egg whites

1½ cups canned pumpkin

½ cup unsweetened applesauce

½ cup water

¾ cup white sugar

¾ cup Splenda

1⅔ cups whole wheat flour

1 teaspoon baking soda

1 teaspoon ground cinnamon

¼ teaspoon ground cloves

¼ teaspoon ground nutmeg

¾ teaspoon salt

¼ teaspoon baking powder

1 tablespoon chopped walnuts

Preheat the oven to 350°F. Coat a 9" × 6" loaf pan with cooking spray and set aside.

Combine the next 6 ingredients in a medium mixing bowl. In a large mixing bowl, combine the baking soda, cinnamon, cloves, nutmeg, salt, flour, and baking powder.

Pour the liquid mixture into the dry mixture and mix well. Pour into the prepared loaf pan and sprinkle the walnuts over the top. Bake for 40 minutes or until a toothpick inserted into the center comes out clean.

Note: *You can also use five mini loaf pans instead of making one large loaf and give the extra loaves away as gifts. Just wrap them in colored plastic wrap and tie with a festive ribbon.*

PROTEIN POWERED	CARBOHYDRATE CONCENTRATED	FAT FRIENDLY	FREE FOODS
Egg whites	Applesauce, sugar, whole wheat flour	Cooking spray, walnuts	Baking soda, cinnamon, cloves, nutmeg, salt, baking powder

CHRISTINE'S NUTRITION NUGGETS This pumpkin bread is a healthy alternative to the typical holiday breads; however, it is not a PC Combo recipe. I often crumble it into my low-fat cottage cheese for a sweet midafternoon PC Combo meal around the holidays. However you choose to eat it, be sure it is paired with a lean protein such as chicken breast, fat-free dairy, or a low-carb protein bar.

Christine's Low-Fat, Low-Sugar Cheesecake

Nutrition facts per serving: 250 calories, 21 grams protein, 27 grams carbohydrates, 6 grams fat SERVES 8

CRUST

1¼ cups graham cracker crumbs

3 tablespoons unsalted butter, melted

¼ cup Splenda

FILLING

2 pounds fat-free cream cheese, softened at room temperature

1¼ cups Splenda

1½ tablespoons fresh lime juice

¼ teaspoon salt

Whites of 6 large eggs

1 cup fresh raspberries

1 cup fat-free whipped topping

Preheat the oven to 350°F.

TO MAKE THE CRUST:

In a medium bowl, combine the graham crackers, melted butter, and Splenda. Place the mixture into a 9" or 6" round cheesecake pan and bake for 10 minutes.

TO MAKE THE FILLING:

In a large bowl, beat the cream cheese and Splenda until smooth. Add the lime juice and salt; continue to beat until smooth. Add the egg whites one at a time, beating after each addition. Pour the filling over the crust and bake for 50 to 60 minutes. Remember to turn the cheesecake halfway through the cooking process. Refrigerate 4 to 6 hours before serving. Top with the raspberries and whipped topping.

PROTEIN POWERED	CARBOHYDRATE CONCENTRATED	FAT FRIENDLY	FREE FOODS
Cream cheese, egg whites	Graham cracker crumbs, raspberries	Butter	Splenda, fat-free whipped topping

CHRISTINE'S NUTRITION NUGGETS This cheesecake is a PC Combo, but that doesn't mean you should eat it on its own. Enjoy this dessert with any dinner from the Skinny Chicks' meal plans by reducing the proteins and carbohydrates to half the suggested portions. Since you get 27 grams of carbohydrates and 21 grams of protein from one slice of this cake, you need to eat only half of your recommended protein and carbs for your main meal.

Pineapple Carpaccio

Nutrition facts per serving: 217 calories, 2 grams protein,
50 grams carbohydrates, 2 grams fat SERVES 4

FRUIT

1 small fresh pineapple, peeled

SYRUP

$1/2$ cup brown sugar

2 cups water

2 cinnamon sticks

1 rosemary sprig

Juice of 2 lemons

1 teaspoon rum extract

1 cup low-fat vanilla ice cream

TO PREPARE THE FRUIT:

Slice the peeled pineapple into thin slices; arrange nicely on four large soup plates.

TO MAKE THE SYRUP:

In a medium saucepan, boil the brown sugar, water, cinnamon sticks, rosemary, lemon juice, and rum extract for 5 minutes. Cover and let set until the syrup returns to room temperature.

Strain using a tea strainer.

Cover the pineapple with the syrup mixture and top with a scoop of vanilla ice cream.

PROTEIN POWERED	CARBOHYDRATE CONCENTRATED	FAT FRIENDLY	FREE FOODS
	Pineapple, brown sugar, vanilla ice cream (8 g carbs per serving)	Low-fat vanilla ice cream (2 g fat per serving)	Cinnamon sticks, rosemary sprig, lemon, rum extract

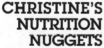

CHRISTINE'S NUTRITION NUGGETS This is a delicious dessert, but it should only be eaten with a low-carb meal because it contains 50 grams of carbs per serving. I enjoy a nice piece of grilled halibut and steamed vegetables for dinner and this pineapple carpaccio for dessert. A meal such as this makes for a delicious and fun PC Combo.

Raspberry Chambord Trifle

Nutrition facts per serving: 315 calories, 21 grams protein,
49 grams carbohydrates, 4 grams fat SERVES 4

16 ounces (4 containers) low-fat (2%) Greek yogurt

2 tablespoons Chambord liqueur

6 tablespoons brown sugar

1 pound fresh raspberries

4 whole mint leaves

4 tablespoons fat-free whipped topping

In a medium bowl, mix the yogurt together with the Chambord and the
brown sugar.

Layer in 4 clear, stemmed glasses, alternating yogurt, then raspberries, then
more yogurt and more raspberries.

Garnish with a mint leaf and whipped topping.

PROTEIN POWERED	CARBOHYDRATE CONCENTRATED	FAT FRIENDLY	FREE FOODS
Low-fat Greek yogurt	Liqueur, brown sugar, raspberries	Low-fat Greek yogurt	Mint leaves, fat-free whipped topping

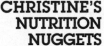 **CHRISTINE'S NUTRITION NUGGETS** This dessert also works as a PC Combo. Feel free to omit the liqueur and serve to your entire family for a fun, delicious snack.

Sautéed California Strawberries

Nutrition facts per serving: 213 calories, 1 gram protein,
52 grams carbohydrates, 0 gram fat SERVES 4

1 pound California strawberries from your favorite farmer's market
Nonstick cooking spray
2 tablespoons turbinado crystal sugar
4 tablespoons aged balsamic vinegar (preferably 20 years old)
1 pint fruit sorbet

Wash the strawberries; stem them and cut in half.

Spray a warm sauté pan with cooking spray.

Add the strawberries and sugar and cook quickly over high heat, until the mixture becomes slightly caramelized, approximately 2 minutes.

Add the vinegar and cook for 1 more minute on high heat.

Serve warm with a scoop of fruit sorbet.

PROTEIN POWERED	CARBOHYDRATE CONCENTRATED	FAT FRIENDLY	FREE FOODS
	Strawberries, sugar, sorbet		Balsamic vinegar

CHRISTINE'S NUTRITION NUGGETS This dessert must be eaten with a low-carb meal, so just swap out the carbs from any meal on the Skinny Chicks plan and enjoy.

Appendix

Food Lists

You can use these lists to create your own meals and for shopping purposes. Remember the portion guidelines:

Proteins: the size of your palm

Carbs: the size of your fist

Fats: the size of a shot glass for nuts and half a shot glass for oils or creams

Kick-Start Plan Foods

PROTEIN

Beef
Organic, preferably grass-fed Filet mignon (beef tenderloin)

Poultry
Chicken breast

Turkey breast

Fish/Shellfish
All types, preferably wild caught

Sushi

Lunchmeat
Low-sodium, fat-free

Chicken

Turkey

Eggs
Eggs, whole (limit 1 per meal)

Egg whites, Eggology 100% pure egg whites, All Whites, Egg Beaters

Cheese
Fat-free and reduced-fat, low-sodium preferred

All flavors and types

String cheese, light (has less fat than the reduced-fat)

Yogurt/Dairy
Plain, fat-free or low-fat

Plain Greek, fat-free or low-fat, flavored fat-free yogurt

Milk, fat-free

Soy milk, light

Vegetarian
Edamame

Lentils

Tofu, low-fat

Protein Powders and Bars
(Use sparingly.)

Egg white protein powder

Whey protein powder

Hemp protein powder

High-protein, high-fiber protein bar

CARBOHYDRATES

Fruits
All types and varieties, fresh or frozen

Pomegranate juice

Pumpkin, canned

Raisins, Dried Apricots, Dates, and Prunes

Vegetables
All types and varieties, fresh, cooked, or frozen; this includes potatoes and yams

Legumes
Black beans, lentils

Grains
Brown rice

Wild rice

Quinoa

Steel-cut oats

Sweetener
Agave nectar

Sugar in the Raw

Honey

Sauces
Enchilada sauce

FATS

Nuts/Seeds
All types, dry roasted or raw

Nut butters

Oils
Extra virgin olive oil

Canola oil

Flaxseed oil

Oil spray/cooking spray

Miscellaneous
Avocado

Black olives

Light mayonnaise

Coconut flakes

Coconut milk, light

Everyday Plan PC Combo Foods

PROTEIN

Beef
Organic, preferably grass-fed

Filet mignon (beef tenderloin)

Poultry
Chicken breast

Turkey breast

Chicken or turkey, ground extra-lean

Turkey jerky

Pork

Canadian bacon, fat-free or low-fat

Fish/Shellfish
All types, preferably wild caught

Sushi

Salmon burger/patty

Lunchmeat
Low-sodium, low-fat

Chicken

Turkey

Eggs
Eggs, whole (limit 1 per meal)

Egg whites, Eggology, All Whites, Egg Beaters

Cheese
Fat-free only, except where indicated in recipe; low-sodium preferred

All flavors and types

String cheese, reduced-fat

Yogurt/Dairy
Plain, fat-free or low-fat

Plain Greek (Voskos brand), fat-free or low-fat

Milk, fat-free

Soy milk, light

Vegetarian
Edamame

Lentils

Seitan

Tempeh

Tofu, low-fat, firm or silken

Veggie burger, low-fat

Veggie slices, low-fat

Veggie dogs, low-fat

Veggie meat, ground, low-fat

Protein Powders and Bars
(Use sparingly) Chocolate, vanilla, strawberry, or plain powder.

Egg white protein powder

Whey protein powder

Hemp protein powder

High-protein, high-fiber protein bar

CARBOHYDRATES

Fruits
All types and varieties, fresh, frozen, or dried

Applesauce, unsweetened

Pomegranate juice

Lemonade

Orange juice

Vegetables
All types and varieties, fresh, cooked, or frozen

Tomato sauce, marinara sauce

Legumes
Black beans

Lentils

Grains
Brown rice

Couscous

Wild rice

Rice pilaf

Quinoa

Polenta

Breads
(Must be whole grain or whole wheat)

Bread

Waffles

Tortillas

Pita

English muffin

Hamburger bun

Bagel

Cereal
Oats, steel-cut or rolled

High-protein cereal

Low-fat granola

Crackers/Snacks
(Whole wheat or whole grain)

Popcorn

Baked chips

Pasta
(Whole wheat or regular)

Noodles, brown rice or regular

Tortillas
Preferably baked

Yellow or white corn

Whole wheat

Yogurt
Flavored, fat-free, all flavors

Sweetener
Agave nectar

Brown sugar

Maple syrup

Sugar in the Raw

Honey

FATS

Nuts/Seeds
All types, dry roasted or raw

Nut butters

Oils
Extra virgin olive oil

Canola oil

Sesame oil

Oil spray/cooking spray

Miscellaneous
Avocado

Black olives

Omega-3 spread

Light mayonnaise

Skinny Chicks Free Foods

You can add these to any meal or eat these foods between meals.

VEGETABLES
**LIMIT 1 C RAW
OR 1/2 C COOKED**

Alfalfa sprouts
Asparagus
Bean sprouts
Bok choy
Broccoli
Cabbage
Cauliflower
Celery
Coleslaw (no dressing)
Collards
Cucumber
Eggplant
Green beans
Kohlrabi
Leek
Lemons and limes
Lettuce, all types
Mustard greens
Okra
Onion
Parsley
Peppers (jalapeño, red, green, bell)
Pickles, dill
Radicchio
Radish
Rutabaga
Sauerkraut
Scallions
Spinach
Squash, summer
Swiss chard
Tomato, raw
Tomato juice
Tomato sauce
Turnip greens
Turnips
Water chestnuts
Watercress
Zucchini

CONDIMENTS
**LIMIT 1 TBSP
PER SERVING**

Apple butter
Balsamic vinegar
Barbecue sauce
Butter Buds
Chicken broth
Cooking spray
Dressing, fat-free
Extracts
Hoisin sauce
Jams, low-sugar
Ketchup
Molly McButter
Mustard (all types)
Parmesan cheese, fat-free
Relish, dill
Rice vinegar
Salsa
Sour cream, fat-free
Soy sauce, low-sodium
Spaghetti sauce
Sriracha chili sauce
Tabasco
Tapatio
Wasabi
White wine vinegar
Worcestershire sauce

BEVERAGES

Coffee, plain, filtered water
Crystal Light drink mixes
Diet Snapple
Hot chocolate, sugar-free
Iced tea (plain/sugar-free)
Seltzer, plain or diet
Soda, diet
Tea, any flavor, unsweetened
Water, filtered or spring
Water, sparkling

HERBS AND SPICES
**ALL HERBS AND SPICES
CAN BE CONSIDERED
FREE; THIS IS A
LIST OF SKINNY CHICKS
FAVORITES**

Bay leaves
Capers
Celery seeds
Chili powder
Chinese spice
Cilantro
Cinnamon
Cloves
Coriander
Curry powder
Garlic (all forms)
Ginger
Ground black pepper
Ground red pepper
Horseradish
Lemon pepper
Mint
Mustard seed
Nutmeg
Paprika
Red-pepper flakes
Rosemary
Saffron
Salt
Thyme
Turmeric
Vanilla bean
White pepper

References

CHAPTER 3

Whitney, Cataldo, Rolfes. "Making Glucose from Protein." *Understanding Normal and Clinical Nutrition,* 2002: 105.

CHAPTER 4

Ludwig, D.S., Majzoub, J.A., Al-Zahrani, A., Dallal, G.E., Blanco, I., and S.B. Roberts. High glycemic index foods, overeating, and obesity. *Pediatrics.* 199; 103E26.

Pawlak, D.B., Kushner, J.A., and D.S. Ludwig. Effects of dietary glycaemic index on adiposity, glucose homeostasis, and plasma lipids in animals. *Lancet.* 2004; 364: 778–85.

CHAPTER 5

Gold, P. et al. Decreases in rat extracellular hippocampal glucose concentration associated with cognitive demands during a spatial task. *Proceedings of the National Academy of Sciences.* 2000; 97(6): 2881–85.

Jenkins, D. et al. Nibbling versus gorging: Metabolic advantage of increased meal frequency. *New England Journal of Medicine.* 1989; 321: 929–34.

Kolata, Gina. "Study Finds that Fat Cells Die and Are Replaced." *The New York Times.* May 5, 2008. Retrieved online May 5, 2008 at http://www.nytimes.com/2008/05/05/health/research/05fat.html?scp-1&sq=Fat+Cell+Die&st=nyt.

CHAPTER 6

Groesz, L. et al. The effect of experimental presentation of thin media images on body satisfaction: A meta-analytic review. *International Journal of Eating Disorders.* 2001; 31(1): 1–16.

CHAPTER 7

Due, A. Effect of normal-fat diets, either medium or high in protein, on body weight in overweight subjects: a randomized 1-year trial. *International Journal of Obesity.* 2004; 18: 1283–90.

Feskanich D., Willett W.C., Stampfer M.J., Colditz G.A. Protein consumption and bone fractures in women. *Am J Epidemiol* 1996; 143: 472–9.

Fittante, Ann, and the Editors of *Prevention* magazine. *The Sugar Solution.* New York: Rodale Inc., 2006.

Halton, T.L., Hu, F.B. The effects of high protein diets on thermogenesis, satiety and weight loss: a critical review. *J Am Coll Nutr* 2004; 23: 373–85.

Sacks, F.M. et al. "Soy Protein, Isoflavones, and Cardiovascular Health." An American Heart Association Science Advisory for Professionals from the Nutrition Committee. *Circulation* 2006.

Vander Wal, J.S. et al. Short-term effect of eggs on satiety in overweight and obese subjects. *Journal of the American College of Nutrition.* 2005; 24(6): 510–15.

Zemel, M. Regulation of adiposity and obesity risk by dietary calcium: Mechanisms and implications. *Journal of the American College of Nutrition.* 2002; 21(2): 146S–151S.

Zemel, M. et al. Calcium and dairy acceleration of weight and fat loss during energy restriction in obese adults. *Obesity Research.* 2004; 12: 582–90.

CHAPTER 8

Feskanich D., Willett W.C., Stampfer M.J., Colditz G.A. Protein consumption and bone fractures in women. *Am J Epidemiol* 1996; 143: 472–9.

Gardner, C.D. et al. Comparison of the Atkins, Zone, Ornish, and LEARN diets for change in weight and related risk factors among overweight premenopausal women: the A TO Z Weight Loss Study: a randomized trial. *Journal of the American Medical Association.* 2007; 297: 969–77.

"Hepatic Encephalopathy." *The New York Times Health Guide.* Retrieved online May 28, 2008 at http://health.nytimes.com/health/guides/disease/hepatic-encephalopathy/overview.html.

Westman, E.C. et al. Effect of 6-month adherence to a very low carbohydrate diet program. *The American Journal of Medicine.* 2002; 113(1): 30–36.

Whitney, Cataldo, Rolfes. "Making Glucose from Protein." *Understanding Normal and Clinical Nutrition,* 2002: 105.

CHAPTER 9

Albert, C. et al. Dietary α-linolenic acid intake and risk of sudden cardiac death and coronary heart disease. *Circulation*. 2005; 112: 3232–38.

Bouchez, Colette. "Want Healthy Skin? Feed It Well." WebMD. Retrieved May 26, 2008 at http://www.webmd.com/skin-problems-and-treatments/features/want-healthy-skin-feed-well

Conklin, S. et al. Serum ω-3 fatty acids are associated with variation in mood, personality and behavior in hypercholesterolemic community volunteers. *Psychiatry Research*. 2007; 152(1): 1–10.

Cromley, Janet. "Eating Away at Illness." *Los Angeles Times*. May 12, 2008. p. R3.

Gallagher, D. et al. Healthy percentage body fat ranges: an approach for developing guidelines based on body mass index. *American Journal of Clinical Nutrition*. 2000; 72(3): 694–701.

Hill, A. et al. Combining fish-oil supplements with regular aerobic exercise improves body composition and cardiovascular disease risk factors. *American Journal of Clinical Nutrition*. 2007; 85(5): 1267–74.

Mozaffarian, D., and E. Rimm. Fish intake, contaminants, and human health: Evaluating the risks and the benefits. *Journal of the American Medical Association*. 2006; 296: 1885–99.

Whitney, et al. "The Economics of Feasting," *Understanding Normal and Clinical Nutrition,* 2002: 221–23.

CHAPTER 10

Brody, Jane. "Personal Health: You Are Also What You Drink." *The New York Times*. March 27, 2007. Retrieved online May 25, 2008 at http://www.nytimes.com/2007/03/27/health/27brody.html.

Cass, D. "Kaiser Permanente Study Shows Alcohol Consumption—No Matter Beverage Type—Linked to Breast Cancer Risk." Sept. 27, 2007. Retrieved online May 26, 2008 at http://ckp.kaiserpermanente.org/newsroom/national/archive/nat_070926_breastcancer.html.

Diepvens, K., Westerterp, K.R., and M.S. Westerterp-Plantega. (2006). Obesity and thermogenesis related to the consumption of caffeine, ephedrine, capsaicin, and green tea. *Am J Physiol Regul Integr Comp Physiol,* July 13; [E-publication ahead of print].

Dulloo, A. et al. Efficiency of green tea extract, polyphenols and caffeine in increasing 24h energy expenditure and fat oxidation in humans. *Am J Clin Nutri,* 1999; 70: 1040–5.

Goulding, Matt. "The 20 Unhealthiest Drinks in America." *Men's Health,* March 2008. Retrieved May 26, 2008 online at http://www.menshealth.com/eathis/Unhealthiest_Drinks_in_America/1_The_Worst_Drink_In_America.php.

Pearson, T. Alcohol and heart disease. *Circulation.* 1996; 94: 3023–35.

Whitney, Cataldo, Rolfes. "Alcohol and Nutrition," *Understanding Normal and Clinical Nutrition,* 2002: 231–33.

Whitney, Cataldo, Rolfes. "Water Losses." *Understanding Normal and Clinical Nutrition,* 2002: 388–89.

CHAPTER 12

Dietary Reference Intakes (DRIs), Food and Nutrition Board, Institute of Medicine, National Academy of Sciences 2004 (from Web site).

CHAPTER 13

Pelletier, C. et al. Associations between weight-loss-induced changes in plasma organochlorine concentrations, serum T3 concentration, and resting metabolic rate. *Toxicological Sciences,* 67 (2002): 46–51.

Turpeinen, J.P. et al. Muscle fiber type I influences lipid oxidation during low-intensity exercise in moderately active middle-aged men. *Scandinavian Journal of Medicine and Science in Sports.* 2006; 16(2): 134–40.

CHAPTER 15

Sohn, Emily. "With Faux Sugars, Real Suspicion." *Los Angeles Times.* Nov. 19, 2007. Retrieved online May 9, 2008 at http://articles.latimes.com/2007/11/19/features/he=sweet19.

APPENDIX

Goel, A. et al. Specific inhibition of cyclooxygenase-2 (COX-2) expression by dietary curcumin in HT-29 human colon cancer cells. *Cancer Lett* 2001 172: 111–18

Kwon, Y.I. et al. Health benefits of traditional corn, beans, and pumpkin: *In vitro* studies for hyperglycemia and hypertension management. *Journal of Medicinal Food.* 2007; 10(2): 266–75.

Acknowledgments

I owe my most special thanks to my husband and most special love, Neil Hazle, my ever-present sounding board, pseudo–writing partner (at many times), and best friend. You truly breathe life into me every day.

An endless thanks and love to all of my clients whose questions, answers, laughter, tears, and completed food journals were the driving force behind this book. You have been my greatest teachers of all.

A huge thank-you to my literary agents, Rusty Robertson and Sue Schwartz. Thanks for standing so firmly behind this book and going above and beyond at every juncture.

For the chance to finally place my life's passion into a book, a sincere thank-you to Nancy Hancock.

An extraordinary, special thanks to Pam Krauss for your extra care and interest in my book and for being the most informative, professional, and wonderful editor I could have ever hoped for. Because of you, this book sings.

To Sharyn Kolberg, your intent listening, understanding, and articulation of my words has been a godsend. You truly blow me away. I'm blessed to have worked with you.

To all the chefs who contributed their amazing recipes to this book. A special thank-you to Chef Denise Macuk for bringing your awesome recipes to my clients and to this book, and to Chef Pierre Sauvaget, whose time and recipes have been invaluable.

My deepest gratitude to my friend and colleague William Smith of INTRAFITT, Inc. Your teaching, prayers, support, and positive energy helped set the blueprint for this book. William, your hard work and knowledge are truly altering the way Americans view weight loss—thank you for all that you do.

To Dr. David Ludwig, for your important work in the area of obesity and for taking the time to discuss your studies with me.

To my dear friend Giuliana Rancic at *E! News*. Besides being an amazing client, you started the ball rolling, and my life has never been the same. After all, you were the one who inspired me to expose those "sinful salads."

A very big thank-you to everyone at Rodale: Beth Lamb, Beth Davey, Zach Greenwald, and the entire group in New York and Pennsylvania for your help and support with the creation of this book.

To the Avanti Nutrition team: Jennifer Williams (junior nutritionist), Gaylie Felchlin (administrative assistant), and Hayley Morrisette (our hardworking intern), your can-do attitudes and teamwork are a blessing. Jen, thanks for being my right hand—you are the best!

To the gals who make me look so good. Melissa Brown is a miracle worker when it comes to beautiful hair—thank you for your amazing work and extreme professionalism. Vivanna Martin of Stila Cosmetics, you are truly heaven sent—thank you for fresh, clean makeup every time!

A loving thanks to my mom, my stepfather Chris, Janine, Lily Zukowski, and Chris Green; you are my biggest heroes, supporters, listeners, and fans. I can't imagine this life without your endless love.

To all my families who have always cheered me on: the Avantis, the Chiminellos, the Seatons, the Surfaces, the Hazles, the Busseys, and the Bybees (especially you, Dad). A big hug to my wonderful aunts Mary, Louise, Gerry, and Sandra. Thanks for your love, encouragement, and neverending prayers. And of course, to my uncle John Chiminello, you are simply the best. Thanks for all your feedback via e-mail.

And most of all, I want to thank my wonderful Lord, Jesus Christ, who is always with me. Thank you for your favor and for taking me to new levels every day.

Index

Boldface page references indicate photographs. <u>Underscored</u> references indicate boxed text.

D

Dairy products, 70, 73, 145. *See also specific type*
Darnit, Get Your Lazy Butt on the Treadmill, 19. *See also* Exercise
Deli meats
  Deli Slices and Fruit, 161
  Low-Sodium Deli Slices and Fruit, 133
  Turkey and Cheese Roll-Up, 131
Delis, eating at, 222–23
Dessert
  California Fruit Kebabs, 280
  Christine's Low-Fat, Low-Sugar Cheesecake, 282
  guidelines, 217
  Low-Fat, Low-Sugar Pumpkin Bread, 281
  Pineapple Carpaccio, 283
  questions about in Skinny Chicks program, 216
  Raspberry Chambord Trifle, 284
  Sautéed California Strawberries, 285
Detoxification, 121, 163
DHA, 98–99, 172
Dietary fat
  "bad," 95–97
  daily intake percentage, 36
  diets low in, 91–92, 99
  energy yields and, 37
  essential fatty acids, 97–99
  in everyday plan guidelines, 136
  glycemic index and, 39
  "good," 97
  importance of, 94–95
  in kick-start plan guidelines, 120
  list of good, 287–88
  monounsaturated, 97
  in nuts, 99–101, 101
  omega-3 fatty acids
    defining, 97–99
    in fish, 72, 143
    health benefits of, 143
    spread, 244
    supplements, 166, 169, 172–73
  omega-6 fatty acids, 97–99
  polyunsaturated, 97
  portion guidelines for, 44
  saturated, 95–96
  "superhero," 97–99
  trans fats, 96
  triglycerides, 69
  weight loss and, 92–94
Dieting
  Atkins diet, 37
  bingeing and, 84
  cabbage soup diet, 37
  drawbacks of, 14
  low- or no-carb diet, 14, 81–83
  low- or no-fat diet, 91–92, 99

magazine articles about, 71, 73
pitfalls, 30–31, 34
starvation theory of, 18, 24–27
Sugar Busters diet, 37
Diners, eating at, 223–24
Dining out
  casual restaurants/dining/takeout, 223–24
  delis, 222–23
  fine dining, 224
  food stands, 222
  increase in, 218–19
  personal account of, 219, 222
Dinner
  Apricot Glazed Chicken with Spicy Quinoa, 269
  Baked Turkey, Sweet Potato, and Steamed Broccoli, 161
  Baked Turkey Chimichanga, 276
  Balsamic Herb Chicken with French Lentils, 271
  Cajun-Style Grilled Shrimp, 133, 268
  Chicken Kebabs on Lemon Grass Skewers, 155, 273
  Christine's Born-Again Lasagna, 153, 262
  Christine's Enchiladas, 149, 277
  Christine's Favorite Steak with Mushroom Sauce, 139, 278–79
  Christine's Pasta and Spicy Red Sauce, 141, 259
  Cilantro Lime Sea Bass, 131, 151, 267
  Citrus Tilapia, 265
  Coconut Curry Sea Bass over Red Lentils, 125, 266
  Creamy Lemon Basil Chicken Linguini, 260
  Grilled Chicken Fajitas with Mango Salsa, 145, 274
  Grilled Halibut with Quinoa and Asparagus, 159
  Grilled White Fish with Quinoa or Brown Rice and Asparagus, 129
  Herb-Crusted Salmon with Baby Potatoes and Artichokes, 127
  Mediterranean Shrimp Pasta, 147, 261
  Mushroom and Artichoke Chicken Scaloppine, 272
  Oven-Roasted Chicken Breast, Rice or Quinoa, Carrots, and Zucchini, 123
  Rosemary-Rubbed Salmon with Brown-Rice and Steamed Artichoke, 163
  Sicilian-Style Chicken and Rice, 165, 270
  skipping, 27
  Smoked Salmon Bagel, 157
  Sugar and Spice Salmon with Barbecue Sweet Potatoes, 264

Mushrooms
  Balsamic Herb Chicken with French
    Lentils, 271
  Christine's Born-Again Lasagna, 153,
    262
  Christine's Favorite Steak with
    Mushroom Sauce, 139, 278–79
  Christine's Pasta and Spicy Red Sauce,
    141, 259
  health benefits of, 270
  Mushroom and Artichoke Chicken
    Scaloppine, 272
  Sicilian-Style Chicken and Rice, 165,
    270
  Veggie Delight Scramble, 132

N

Nectarines
  Deli Slices and Fruit, 161
  High-Fiber, Low-Fat Protein Bar and
    Fruit, 123
  Low-Sodium Deli Slices and Fruit, 133
Negative thinking, 54–57
Nutrition
  balance of blood sugar levels and, 43
  challenge of, 14
  defining, 42–43
  effects of lack of, 25, 26
  health and, 45
  for meal plans, 120
  PC Combo and, 45
  Skinny Chicks program and, 37
Nuts
  Apple Maple Pecan Parfait, 138
  Blueberry Yogurt Parfait with Slivered
    Almonds, 150
  California Fruit Kebabs, 280
  dietary fat in, 99–101, 101
  Greek Yogurt with Honey and Walnuts,
    163
  Honey Nut Apple Crunch, 158
  Low-Fat, Low-Sugar Pumpkin Bread,
    281
  Maple Walnut Ricotta Bake, 246
  protein in, 100–101, 101
  satiety and, 101

O

Oat flour, 246
Oats
  Apple Raisin Oatmeal, 156
  Berry Delish Oatmeal, 146
  Cinnamon Raisin Oatmeal Muffins, 242
  fiber in, 135
  Steel-Cut Oats with Side of Sweet
    Yogurt, 134
Obesity epidemic, 31, 109
Oils, 120, 161
Olive oil, 161

Olives
  Baked Chips and Cheesy Salsa, 152
  Christine's Enchiladas, 149, 277
  Citrus Tilapia, 265
  health benefits of, 265
Oranges
  Citrus Tilapia, 265
  Citrus-y Greek Yogurt, 127
  juice, 38, 42
  Mandarin, 252
  Thai Chicken Lettuce Cups, 252
Overeating, 30

P

Pasta
  brown rice noodles, 263
  Christine's Born-Again Lasagna, 153,
    262
  Christine's Pasta and Spicy Red Sauce,
    141, 259
  Creamy Lemon Basil Chicken Linguine,
    260
  image of, 65–66
  Mediterranean Shrimp Pasta, 147, 261
  Sicilian Chicken Soup, 254
  Wasabi Sesame Salmon with Brown Rice
    Noodles, 143, 263
PC Combo
  blood sugar levels and, 37, 39
  carbohydrates and, 89
  Christine's Low-Fat, Low-Sugar
    Cheesecake and, 282
  in everyday plan guidelines, 136
  food list, 288
  in kick-start plan guidelines, 119
  nutrition and, 45
  Pineapple Carpaccio and, 283
  protein and, 67
  Raspberry Chambord Trifle and, 284
  Skinny Chicks program and, 67, 89
  in vegetarian diet, 74
  weight loss and, 68
Peaches
  Blueberry Peach Smoothie, 130
  Deli Slices and Fruit, 161
  Low-Sodium Deli Slices and Fruit, 133
  Tuna-Stuffed Celery Sticks with Fruit,
    128
Peanut butter
  Baked Yam Stuffed with Peanut Butter,
    Cottage Cheese, and Cinnamon,
    124
  Chocolate Peanut Butter Smoothie,
    162
  Peanut Butter Toast, 144
  Thai Chicken Lettuce Cups, 252
Pears
  High-Fiber, Low-Fat Protein Bar with
    Anjou Pear, 155